THE CONCISE GUIDE TO
Bipolar Disorder

THE CONCISE GUIDE TO
Bipolar Disorder

Francis Mark Mondimore, MD

Johns Hopkins University Press

Baltimore

Note to the Reader: This book is not meant to substitute for medical care, and treatment should not be based solely on its contents. Instead, treatment must be developed in a dialogue between the individual and their physician. This book has been written to help with that dialogue.

Drug dosage: The author and publisher have made reasonable efforts to determine that the selection of drugs discussed in this text conform to the practices of the general medical community. The medications described do not necessarily have specific approval by the US Food and Drug Administration for use in the diseases for which they are recommended. In view of ongoing research, changes in governmental regulation, and the constant flow of information relating to drug therapy and drug reactions, the reader is urged to check the package insert of each drug for any change in indications and dosage and for warnings and precautions. This is particularly important when the recommended agent is a new and / or infrequently used drug.

© 2022 Johns Hopkins University Press
All rights reserved. Published 2022
Printed in the United States of America on acid-free paper
2 4 6 8 9 7 5 3 1

Johns Hopkins University Press
2715 North Charles Street
Baltimore, Maryland 21218-4363
www.press.jhu.edu

Library of Congress Cataloging-in-Publication Data

Names: Mondimore, Francis Mark, 1953– author.
Title: The concise guide to bipolar disorder / Francis Mark Mondimore, MD.
Description: Baltimore : Johns Hopkins University Press, 2022. | Includes
  bibliographical references and index.
Identifiers: LCCN 2021039029 | ISBN 9781421443898 (hardcover) | ISBN
  9781421444031 (paperback) | ISBN 9781421444048 (ebook)
Subjects: LCSH: Manic-depressive illness —Popular works. | Manic-depressive
  illness —Treatment —Popular works.
Classification: LCC RC516 .M635 2022 | DDC 616.89/5 —dc23
LC record available at https:// lccn.loc.gov/ 2021039029

A catalog record for this book is available from the British Library.

Special discounts are available for bulk purchases of this book.
For more information, please contact Special Sales at specialsales@jh.edu.

Contents

What Causes Bipolar Disorder? 171

Putting It All Together 199

Preface

You or a loved one has recently been diagnosed with bipolar disorder, and you want some information *now*. You may be thinking, "I can't handle too much detail just yet, but I need to understand the basics—and *fast*." I wrote this book for you.

• Part I will tell you what you need to know about the illness itself: its symptoms, the different forms it can take, and how psychiatrists diagnose bipolar disorder.

• Part II will tell you about treatments. There are chapters on the different types of medications we prescribe. I will discuss a group of treatment interventions that together are called *brain stimulation treatments*. These treatments use tiny electrical impulses to stimulate brain areas. Next, I'll discuss the different types of psychotherapy, including talk therapy, which is such an essential aspect of treatment.

• Part III lays out what *you* can do to stay well. This includes lifestyle changes and healthy habits that research has shown can help minimize symptoms and maximize healthy time. I'll discuss how to prepare for emergencies and also share recommendations especially meant for family members.

• Part IV is about the causes of bipolar disorder and discusses how treatments work. Its content is more "scientific," and these chapters may be considered optional reading. However, I urge you not to skip them. It's a lot easier to put your treatment team's recommendations into place if you know a little about the science behind them.

• Part V is a short chapter that looks ahead and discusses research into the illness's causes and the quest for new and better treatments.

About two percent of the population suffers from some form of bipolar disorder. If that statistic is broadened, however, to include milder forms of the illness, known as *soft* bipolar conditions, then that number rises to nearly five percent.

Clinical research has shown again and again that many relapses of bipolar disorder occur not because of medication failure but rather because people stop taking medication and drop out of treatment. Perhaps they don't understand that relapse and repetition of illness episodes are hallmarks of the disease, that *abruptly* stopping medication is especially risky, that medication side effects can often be treated or controlled, and that new medicines are becoming available all the time. I hope this book helps those who face difficult treatment decisions to make well-informed and intelligent choices.

A survey of individuals with bipolar disorder and other mood disorders, carried out by the National Depressive and Manic-Depressive Association (now known as the Depression and Bipolar Support Alliance) in the early 1990s, found that thirty-six percent of those who responded to the survey had not sought professional treatment until more than *ten years* after their symptoms had begun. Of the people with bipolar disorder in this study, seventy-three percent had received at least one incorrect diagnosis before being identified as having bipolar disorder—often many years after first seeking help. The average respondent had seen 3.3 physicians before being correctly diagnosed. Another study, done in 2017, showed only a small improvement in the length of time it took people with bipolar disorder to get into treatment: the number of years had dropped from ten to just under six.

Why is this illness so difficult to identify correctly? One reason is that the most severe form of the illness—called bipolar I disorder—is both easily diagnosed and just one of the several forms this chameleon disorder can take. Bipolar I, in fact, is probably less common than the milder forms, in which symptoms of mild depression and subtle "mood swings" may be the only manifestations. We are realizing that many people with these milder forms of the disorder also benefit from treatment with mood-stabilizing medications. But they can do so only when they seek treatment and are correctly diagnosed.

Winston Churchill, George Frideric Handel, Lord Byron, Virginia Woolf, Edgar Allan Poe, Napoleon Bonaparte, and Vincent van Gogh are a few of the politicians, writers, artists, and musicians who, despite having bipolar disorder, left their mark of greatness upon the world. In our own time, musical sensation Mariah Carey, *Star Wars* actress Carrie Fisher, and television anchor and journalist Jane Pauley have acknowledged being diagnosed with bipolar disorder. The list could go on and on.

Most people who are affected by this illness, however, are just ordinary human beings who want nothing more than to get back to their everyday lives after they or their family members have been diagnosed with the disorder.

By picking up this book, you have already taken an essential step toward getting better and staying well—or helping your loved one do so. Numerous research studies have shown that people who get educated about the illness do better. They have fewer relapses, spend less time struggling with symptoms, and have higher social and occupational functioning levels. By facing the illness straight on and deciding to learn about it, you have already increased your chances of doing well. *Congratulations!*

PART I

What Is Bipolar Disorder?

❖ **Bipolar disorder is a *mood disorder.***
Chapter 1 answers some basic questions like "What is *mood?*" and "What is *normal* mood?" It then describes the types of abnormal mood states that people with bipolar disorder experience. You'll hear from some individuals who will describe their experiences of abnormal mood states. It's important to know beforehand that not everyone with bipolar disorder will experience all the symptoms this chapter describes. Every person's experience of bipolar disorder is unique. There are many variations in the types of symptoms an individual will have and the severity of their symptoms.

❖ **There are several subtypes of bipolar disorder. The illness is classified according to the types and duration of symptoms that the person experiences.**
Chapter 2 describes how this classification system works and discusses how psychiatrists make the diagnosis. You will also learn that this system is not perfect. There are many individuals whose illness doesn't fit into neat categories. You'll learn why the condition can be so challenging to diagnose and why many cases of "depression" turn out to be a form of bipolar disorder.

CHAPTER 1

Normal and Abnormal Mood

Bipolar disorder is a *mood disorder,* a psychiatric illness that causes problems with mood regulation.

Mood

Mood is a collection of feelings that make up our basic sense of mental and physical well-being. It includes feelings such as happiness or sadness, optimism or pessimism. It also includes physical sensations such as fatigue or vigor. Our mood is essentially our emotional temperature, a whole set of feelings that expresses emotional comfort or discomfort.

When people are in a good mood, they are confident and optimistic, relaxed and friendly, patient, interested, content. People in a good mood feel energetic and have a sense of physical well-being. They sleep soundly and eat heartily. It's easy for them to socialize and be affectionate. The future looks bright and the time ripe for starting new projects. When we're in a good mood, the world seems like a wonderful place. It feels good to be alive.

When we're in a low mood, an opposite set of feelings takes over. We turn inward and are preoccupied or distracted by our thoughts. There may be a sense of emptiness and loss. It can be challenging to think about the future. When we do, it's hard not to be pessimistic or even intimidated. We lose our temper more quickly and then feel guilty about it. It's difficult to be sociable, so we avoid others and prefer to be alone. Energy is low. Self-doubt takes over; we become preoccupied and worry about how other people see us.

Usually, our mood changes with our situation and circumstances. However, in people with bipolar disorder, a person's moods go up and down on their own, with little relationship to what is going on in the individual's life. People with bipolar disorder suffer from more extreme "ups" and more profound "lows." Also, these abnormal mood states often go on for long periods of time. Abnormally high or abnormally low moods can last for weeks, months, or even years at a time.

Psychiatrists have defined and described four types of abnormal mood states in bipolar disorder. People with the illness cycle into and out of one or more of these abnormal states during the course of their illness.

Mania

Mania is a state of abnormally high or irritable mood and is the most extreme and dramatic of the symptom clusters of bipolar disorder. In the manic state, the mood regulator switches into "high" (table 1.1). Many people who have bipolar disorder never have a full-blown manic episode, but a manic episode makes the diagnosis of bipolar disorder certain.

Mania often starts gradually and may take weeks to develop fully. In the early stages, the mood state slowly moves "upward," and people find themselves filled with pleasant feelings of vitality. This heightened sense of well-being and confidence grows and gradually evolves into euphoria.

Changes in thinking accompany the mood changes. The individual feels that they are thinking more clearly and more rationally than usual. A feeling that mental processes are moving *faster* than usual also develops. At first, there may be only a pleasant sense of quickness of thinking. Invariably, however, thinking processes accelerate: "quick" becomes "fast" and finally "racing." Racing

Table 1.1. Symptoms of mania

Mood symptoms
Elated, euphoric mood
Irritable mood
Grandiosity

Cognitive (thinking) symptoms
Feelings of heightened concentration
Accelerated thinking ("racing thoughts")

Bodily symptoms
Increased energy level
Decreased need for sleep
Erratic appetite
Increased libido

Symptoms of psychosis
Grandiose delusions
Hallucinations

thoughts are a symptom so typical of mania that the diagnosis becomes doubtful if this symptom is absent. This tumbling, jumbled jumping from one thought to another becomes progressively worse and more unpleasant as the episode develops.

As the individual's manic thinking speeds up, their speech does as well. Rapid, or *pressured*, speech (the term usually used by psychiatrists) is nearly always seen in mania. People experiencing mania speak more and more quickly as the episode develops, trying to express the ideas whirling through their consciousness at ever-faster speeds. Sometimes racing thoughts and pressured speech lead to an outpouring of furious writing, page after incomprehensible page of it.

Their increased energy and confidence push people having a manic episode into rising levels of activity. They start new, often

In Their Own Words: Mania

"At this point, I hadn't slept for five days. The longer I stayed up, the more powerful I became . . . I drank beer, I smoked pot, and did shots with drunks. I latched onto any girl willing to listen to me. After everyone went to sleep, I took long walks while listening to my Walkman and thinking about the universe. I always brought a notebook to make sure I captured my great ideas on paper. My thoughts would flow faster than I could write . . . [A]s soon as I got a good one, I wanted to act on it. A strong belief that telepathic communication would rule the future recurred over and over and I tried to read the minds of passersby. I knew it would take time to master the art of telepathy, but I was prepared for the long haul."

Peter J. Barnes, *Sixty Days to Sanity: A College Freshman's Struggle to Overcome Mental Illness* (Printed by the author, 2005), 30.

unrealistic projects and suddenly develop new interests in matters that never interested them before. They may act on sudden urges to travel, learn new languages, play a musical instrument. Whatever the new pursuit is, the person with mania throws themselves into it 110 percent, spending hours on end on some new project or staying up all night working.

The high feelings that characterize mania cause a loss of inhibitions. This can result in spending sprees, sexual promiscuity, and the overuse of alcohol and other intoxicating substances. The spending sprees can be extravagant and financially catastrophic because the person with mania has no concern for where the money will come from to pay the bills.

There are almost always changes in sleeping and eating habits in mania. A decreased need for sleep is one of the first symptoms to develop—often a clue for individuals who have been manic before that another episode may be starting. Food intake is usually reduced because people in a manic episode simply don't have time to eat. The subsequent weight loss can be dramatic.

As the combination of euphoric mood and mental quickness develops, the individual with mania begins to feel tremendously self-confident, the so-called *grandiosity* of the manic state. Fears of unpleasant consequences disappear, and reckless enthusiasm takes over. The affected person may seek out new adventures and experiences with no regard for the possible adverse repercussions. They can begin to lose touch with reality and start *believing* in the great things they feel capable of doing. A fantastic, indescribable feeling of mental power and significance takes over. People with mania can develop *grandiose delusions*. They can become convinced that they are the president or prime minister, a scientific genius, or a modern prophet. They may feel called upon to found a new religion. They may even believe they are the reincarnation of Christ or possibly a new god.

The "feeling good" stage of mania is sometimes very short-lived. An angry, irritable mood can quickly replace the initially elevated mood. Sometimes the individual in a manic state alternates between elation and irritability for a time, but usually the irritable, unpleasant mood becomes predominant. It is often this irritability that brings the person to the attention of medical professionals.

As the manic state continues to develop, racing thoughts, an increased energy level, and loss of inhibitions lead to disorganized and disturbed thinking and behavior. People in this state become incoherent and agitated. At this point, the manic state is not pleasant—even if it may have started that way. The full-blown manic state is not only intensely unpleasant but also dangerous. The danger may arise from the increased risk of violence toward others (or toward themselves) and the physical stress the syndrome causes. In decades past, mania had a significant mortality rate. People with mania died in a state of progressive exhaustion, dehydration, and cardiovascular collapse.

Major Depression

Major depression is a state of profound low mood accompanied by impairments in thinking and memory, the loss of the ability to enjoy usually pleasurable activities, disturbances of sleep and appetite, physical and mental sluggishness or agitation, and, frequently, suicidal thinking and behavior (table 1.2). Nearly all people with bipolar disorder go through periods of major depression. For most, major depression dominates their illness. Of their abnormal mood states, they spend substantially more time in a depressed state than in a manic one.

The mood of major depression is a relentless, pervasive gloom that continues from one day to the next and from which the afflicted person cannot rouse themself. Individuals with depression find their thinking dominated by thoughts of sadness and loss, regret and hopelessness. Guilty ruminations are especially characteristic, and psychiatrists often make a particular point to ask about guilty feelings when they evaluate a person for depression. Ruminations about guilt, shame, and regret are typical in the depressed states of mood disorders. However, they are very *uncommon* in the "normal" depressed mood. People experiencing the normal depressed mood that comes after a personal loss attribute their bad feelings to the fact that a loss has occurred. Only in unusual circumstances will they believe that they are to blame for their problem and feel guilty or ashamed. However, the individual having a major depressive episode frequently thinks that they are to blame for their troubles—and sometimes for other people's troubles as well. The presence of guilty preoccupations is a significant sign of clinical depression.

Many people with major depression do not describe their depressed mood as "sad" because they instead have a tense, miserable sort of mood called *dysphoria*. This fact makes the critical point that major depression is *not* simply an exaggeration of an ordinary low mood that may be a reaction to disappointment or loss.

Table 1.2. Symptoms of depression

Mood symptoms

Depressed mood
Dysphoric, tense miserable mood
Diurnal variation of mood (early-morning depression,
   mood improving as day goes on)
Guilty feelings
Loss of ability to feel pleasure (anhedonia)
Social withdrawal
Suicidal thoughts

Bodily symptoms

Sleep disturbance
  • insomnia
  • hypersomnia
Appetite disturbance
  • weight loss
  • weight gain
Loss of interest in sex
Fatigue
Constipation
Headaches
Worsening of painful conditions

Cognitive (thinking) symptoms

Poor concentration
Poor memory
Indecision
Slowed thinking

Symptoms of psychosis

Delusional thinking
Hallucinations
Catatonic states

"Depression" or "DEPRESSION"?

A colleague of mine likes to talk about the differences between depression "with a little *d*" as opposed to "big *D*" depression. She refers to the kind of normal, expected low mood that everyone experiences from time to time as (little *d*) depression and the clinical syndrome described in this section as (big *D*) Depression, or, better yet, DEPRESSION. The feelings that people with mood disorders experience when they are in a depressed (make that DEPRESSED) episode are *not* simply exaggerations of the universal human experience of normal sadness.

Another core feature of major depression is the loss of interest in usually pleasurable activities. The person who is depressed cannot derive any pleasure from listening to music, going to a movie, or engaging in the sports or hobbies that usually provide enjoyment. This loss of the ability to feel pleasure has come to be called *anhedonia* (derived from the Greek word for "pleasure").

Energy level and thinking are also affected—in an opposite direction of polarity from that seen in mania. The person with depression experiences a slowing and inefficiency in thinking and a feebleness of memory and concentration. Information processing and reasoning falter, and simple decisions can become overwhelming dilemmas. In the elderly, these sorts of thinking problems can be so severe that depression is misdiagnosed as Alzheimer's disease.

Severe depression almost always causes a change in sleeping patterns. People with depression frequently have insomnia, but may also experience its opposite, sleeping too much (*hypersomnia* is the technical term). In the depression associated with bipolar disorder, oversleeping seems especially common—perhaps more common than in other types of clinical depression, where insomnia is more common.

Appetite is also usually disturbed in individuals with depression. As with sleep problems, changes occur in both directions, and people may eat too much or too little. They may lose or gain a significant amount of weight during periods of depression. As might be expected, the person with depression loses interest in sex, a symptom best understood as part of the person's inability to experience pleasurable activities of any kind.

One of the most common bodily symptoms that occurs in depression is a sense of fatigue, with prominent low energy and listlessness. Headaches, constipation, and a feeling of heaviness in the chest are also common, as are other, more difficult to describe sensations of physical discomfort. People who have preexisting painful medical conditions such as arthritis or inflammatory bowel disease are usually more bothered by the symptoms of these illnesses when depressed. Connections between depression and problems with the fatigue seen in chronic fatigue immunodeficiency syndrome and the painful joint and muscle disease fibromyalgia are well described in the research literature, but they are poorly understood. Depression seems to lower the pain threshold: individuals with depression are more sensitive to pain and are more distressed by it.

In Their Own Words: Major Depression

"My indecisiveness was the worst of all. I couldn't decide what to eat or what to wear. I couldn't decide whether to get out of bed or to stay. I couldn't decide whether to shower or not to shower. I could never decide what to do because I didn't know myself."

Norman Endler, *Holiday of Darkness: A Psychologist's Personal Journey Out of His Depression* (New York: John Wiley and Sons, 1982), 4.

Just as in the syndrome of mania, people suffering through an episode of the depression of bipolar disorder can experience distortions of thinking that psychiatrists call *delusions*. As their view of the world and of themselves becomes increasingly colored by their pervasive mood changes, individuals with depression can come to believe that terrible things are happening all around them, that they will be fired from their job or lose a professional license or certification, and that their family will become destitute. In addition to such *delusions of poverty*, delusions can arise from the uncomfortable physical sensations of depression. They may believe they have cancer, AIDS, or some other life-threatening illness.

Hallucinations occur in severe depression but not as frequently as in mania. The hallucinations are consistent with the mood and are frightening, even horrifying. Emil Kraepelin, the early twentieth-century German psychiatrist who published the first textbook on what we now call bipolar disorder, described his patients' hallucinations: "[They] see evil spirits, death . . . crowds of monsters . . . dead relatives. . . . The patient hears his tortured relatives

---

In Their Own Words: Major Depression

"I had now reached that phase of the disorder where all sense of hope had vanished, along with the idea of futurity; my brain . . . had become less an organ of thought than an instrument registering, minute by minute, varying degrees of its own suffering . . . I'd feel the horror, like some poisonous fog bank, roll in upon my mind, forcing me to bed. There I would lie for as long as six hours, stuporous and virtually paralyzed, gazing at the ceiling."

William Styron, *Darkness Visible: A Memoir of Madness* (New York: Random House, 1990), 19.

screaming and lamenting. . . . His food tastes of soapy water or excrement, of corpses and mildew."

Some seriously ill people sink into a state of lethargy and despair that is called *depressive stupor.* In an era when virtually no treatment was available for this terrible condition, Kraepelin described this deepest abyss of depression: "The patients lie in bed taking no interest in anything. They betray no pronounced emotion; they are mute, inaccessible. They pass their [bowel movements] under them; they stare straight in front of them with [a] vacant expression . . . like a mask and with wide-open eyes." Fortunately, modern psychiatrists only rarely see a patient depressed to this point, a condition called *catatonia.*

Hypomania

Hypomania is a state of abnormally elevated mood, increased activity, and decreased need for sleep, similar to mania but without the mental disorganization and behavioral disturbances seen in people with mania. Hypomania can be thought of as the symptoms present only at the beginning of a manic episode: the elated mood, increased energy level, rapid thinking and speaking, and sometimes a bit of irritability.

People in the hypomanic state do not have the severe mental disorganization of mania. They are by definition not agitated to the point of violence toward themselves or others. Nevertheless, hypomania can have unpleasant consequences. Feelings of increased confidence can lead to foolish investments in real estate or the stock market. They can squander personal resources on grandiose and risky business ventures. Increased sexual feelings can lead to extramarital affairs. Irritability can lead to arguments and disagreements with family, colleagues, or neighbors that can sour relationships, sometimes permanently. Even people with mild hypomania can quit a good job in a burst of overconfidence or withdraw their life savings for a get-rich-quick scheme. They may simply begin to drive their car too fast. All these behaviors can have devastating consequences.

In Their Own Words: Hypomania

"Most of the time I was busy, busy, busy; taping records, playing tennis, skiing, writing manuscripts, talking . . . reading, going to movies, staying up at night, waking up early in the morning, always on the go—busy, busy, busy . . . As a hypomanic, I didn't stop to analyze my thoughts, feelings, or behavior. I was much too busy and didn't always stop to think about what I was doing . . . I was critical of others and occasionally told some people off publicly . . . I was aggressive, talked incessantly, and interrupted others while they were speaking."

Norman Endler, *Holiday of Darkness: A Psychologist's Personal Journey Out of His Depression* (New York: John Wiley and Sons, 1982), 4.

Individuals in a hypomanic state rarely seek treatment, at least initially—remember, they are feeling *quite* well. After some time of living with the illness, however, many people recognize that hypomania—as wonderful as it feels at the time—is usually a sign of trouble. It may presage a crash into depression or further escalation into mania.

Because individuals in a hypomanic state are *not* psychotic, they often cannot be involuntarily treated for their illness. This is because the criteria for involuntary treatment insist upon "dangerous" behaviors. People who are hypomanic can avoid treatment for weeks, even months, consequently ruining their financial status, credit rating, employment history, relationships, and health.

As we shall see later in this chapter, some people with bipolar disorder experience episodes of depression and hypomania but never develop full-blown mania. This is one reason why the term *manic-depressive illness* was dropped from the psychiatric vocabulary many decades ago. The classic "manic-depressive" disorder—

episodes of full-blown mania and major depression—may be only one of many forms of the illness.

Mixed Mood States

Mixed mood states (sometimes called "mixed affective states") are abnormal mood states that combine the features of both depression and mania/hypomania. Other labels used for the mixed state are *mixed mania* and *dysphoric mania*.

Psychiatrists do not yet agree on this mood state's defining characteristics, but they have long recognized that symptoms of depression and mania seem to exist almost simultaneously in some people (table 1.3). This state represents a distinct variety of abnormal moods, separate from depression and typical mania but combining features of both. The accelerated thinking and hyperactivity typical of the manic state remain its most striking features. Instead of a euphoric mood, these changes become combined with a depressed, despairing, desperate mood.

Just as full-blown mania is unmistakable, so is a full-blown mixed state. But in the same way that a state of mild hypomania can be challenging to distinguish from an elevated but normal

Table 1.3. Symptoms of a mixed mood state in ten patients

Symptoms	Percentage of patients
Depressed mood	100
Irritable mood	100
Increased activity	100
Insomnia	93
Pressured speech	93
Hostility	79
Flight of ideas	43
Anxiety attacks	43
Delusions (depressive)	36
Delusions (nondepressive)	21

Source: Data from Frederick K. Goodwin and Kay Redfield Jamison, *Manic-Depressive Illness* (New York: Oxford University Press, 1990), 49.

mood, mild mixed states can be difficult to recognize. A mild mixed state sometimes lasts only a few hours. Whenever a patient tells me about being troubled by uncomfortable, angry "rages," I suspect that they may be having mild mixed states. *Anxiety* is another word that people often use to describe their experience of this mood state. However, it is not the fearful fretfulness of ordinary anxiety; this state is more like a pressure cooker full of depressed emotions, ready to explode.

The mixed state can be dangerous because the individual has negative, depressing thought patterns together with excess energy, restlessness, and an inner sense of pressure and tension. This negative energy puts people in mixed states at high risk for hurting themselves with suicidal behaviors. And it is often while in a mixed state that individuals engage in a variety of self-destructive behaviors that are not immediately life-threatening. They may cut or burn themselves. Patients have told me that desperate behav-

---

In Their Own Words: Mixed Mood States

"On occasion, these periods of total despair would be made even worse by terrible agitation. My mind would race from subject to subject, but instead of being filled with the exuberance and cosmic thoughts that had been associated with earlier periods of rapid thinking, it would be drenched in awful sounds and images of decay and dying; dead bodies on the beach, charred remains of animals, toe-tagged corpses in morgues. During these agitated periods, I became exceedingly restless, angry, and irritable, and the only way I could dilute the agitation was to run along the beach or pace back and forth across my room like a polar bear at the zoo."

Kay Redfield Jamison, *An Unquiet Mind: A Memoir of Moods and Madness* (New York: Vintage Books, 1996), 36.

iors like these help them shift a terrible inner pain and tension from "inside" to "the outside." For them, physical pain is somehow easier to deal with than a mixed state's painful agitation.

Key Takeaways

❖ *Bipolar disorder is a mood disorder, a psychiatric illness that causes problems with mood regulation.*

❖ *There are four types of abnormal mood states in bipolar disorder that have been defined and described by psychiatrists: mania, major depression, hypomania, and mixed states. People with bipolar disorder cycle into and out of one or more of these abnormal states during the course of their illness.*

CHAPTER 2

Types of Bipolar Disorder

Bipolar disorder is classified into several types depending on which mood states are present during the patient's illness. Three of these types—*bipolar I, bipolar II,* and *cyclothymic disorder*—are well defined. There is disagreement about how to classify the many other variations of the illness that can occur. These are usually lumped together in a category called "soft" bipolar disorders.

Bipolar I Disorder

People with *bipolar I disorder* have full-blown manic attacks and deep, paralyzing depressions. In a World Health Organization survey of more than sixty-one thousand people in eleven countries, the prevalence rate of bipolar I disorder was 0.6 percent. This means that about six in one thousand people suffer from bipolar I disorder. Bipolar I disorder usually starts in late adolescence or early adulthood, with the peak onset during the third decade of life (ages 20 through 29).

A schematic representation of the moods of bipolar I appears in figure 2.1. The pattern of abnormal mood episodes seems to vary widely, and the rhythm of the illness is almost as individual as the patient who has it.

Bipolar I is often a relapsing and remitting illness, meaning that its symptoms come and go. This feature of bipolar I—and it is a feature of *all* mood disorders—makes it challenging to diagnose, challenging to treat, and fiendishly difficult to study.

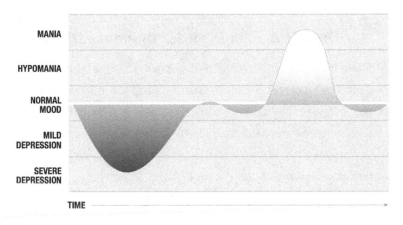

MANIA

HYPOMANIA

NORMAL
MOOD

MILD
DEPRESSION

SEVERE
DEPRESSION

TIME

Figure 2.1. Mood changes in bipolar I. *Source: Illustration by Jenna Macfarlane.*

Bipolar I: What to Expect

Many excellent clinical studies about bipolar disorder were done in the years before effective treatments were available. These studies document and illustrate the pattern of symptoms that occurs if bipolar disorder is not treated what physicians call the *natural history* of the illness.

How many episodes of illness did people have in the days before treatment was available? How long did their episodes last? What was the length of time between episodes?

In a 1942 study, researchers looked at the medical records of sixty-six patients with "manic-depressive psychosis." Some had records available for up to twenty-six years. A few patients had only one episode of illness in the study period. About one-third had two to three episodes, about one-third had four to six episodes, and about one-third had more than seven (table 2.1). A few had twenty or more episodes. Unfortunately, there is no way to know whether the individual will have another two or three episodes during their lifetime or more than twenty.

In this study, the average duration of mood episodes was about six and a half months. Still, depressions and manias can be shorter or sometimes last much longer. In the days before modern treatment, people could be in a manic state for years. Fortunately,

How Is Bipolar Disorder Diagnosed?

There is at present no blood test or brain scan that can diagnose bipolar disorder. Psychiatrists make a diagnosis by gathering information from the patient about *family history* and the types and patterns of *symptoms*.

The patient's *family history* is essential to consider because bipolar disorder is known to run in families— that is, the illness has a substantial genetic component. Of all the risk factors for developing this illness, genetic influences account for over half. A 2019 Swedish study of twins calculated that the percentage of the risk attributable to genetic factors (a number called the *heritability* of the illness) is sixty percent. This means that if a person seeking treatment for mood symptoms has a family member who has been diagnosed with bipolar disorder, the chances that they also have bipolar disorder are significantly increased.

You've already read about the *symptoms* that characterize the manic state, hypomania, major depression, and mixed states. Full-blown manic states are unmistakable, as is major depression. Hypomania can be more difficult to ferret out because people who have had hypomanic periods often do not recognize them as abnormal. Therefore, they do not think to report them when asked about mood. The psychiatrist must know to ask about periods of high energy, decreased need for sleep, and elevated moods that seem to come and go of their own accord. Frequently, family members of the affected person notice these periods even if the person who had them does not. This is one reason why a psychiatrist will often ask a new patient to bring a family member to the evaluation appointment. Alternatively, they may ask for permission to call a family member to get information from another observer.

As you will see in this section, the *pattern* of symptoms is what determines the type of bipolar disorder that gets diagnosed. Again, family members can be invaluable sources for this type of information.

The psychiatrist will ask about other details of the patient's experiences suggesting a bipolar diagnosis. For example, many medications can trigger manic or hypomanic symptoms or just make a person with bipolar disorder feel over-energized or agitated. Antidepressants are the most common culprits in this regard, but steroid medications and stimulant medications, such as methylphenidate, have been implicated as well.

modern psychiatrists no longer see patients who are manic for years at a time. Effective current treatments bring these episodes to a close, and the patient is usually better in a few days—weeks at most.

How about the time between attacks? For many people with bipolar disorder, modern treatments are quite effective at keeping the episodes from recurring. But how long did remissions last in the days before these treatments were available? Emil Kraepelin noted that the time between episodes could be years, even decades—in one case, forty-four years passed between one episode of illness and the next.

Subsequent studies have shown that, if untreated, episodes of

Table 2.1. Number of episodes of illness in sixty-six patients with
bipolar disorder

Number of episodes	Percentage of patients
1	8
2–3	29
4–6	26
More than 7	37

Source: Data from Thomas A. C. Rennie, "Prognosis in Manic-Depressive
Psychoses," *American Journal of Psychiatry* 98, no. 6 (1942): 801–14. https://doi
.org/10.1176/ajp.98.6.801.
Note: This study was done before any treatments were available for bipolar disorder.

bipolar disorder often occur more frequently as people age and
seem to be triggered more easily.

Another finding in these studies is that many people "switch"
from a depression to a manic episode with no normal mood interval. Many individuals have a period of depression lasting several weeks or months and then switch into a manic episode, again
of several months' duration. Often there is another switch, and
a third phase of the episode sets in: a long period of depression
(figure 2.2).

A 1969 study described the course of one hundred manic
episodes and also noted the relationship of manic to depressed
periods. In this study, about half of the patients' manic episodes
showed at least one switch—a depression either before or after a
manic episode. There is some evidence that people who "switch"
from depression to mania have a more difficult-to-treat form of
the illness than those who switch from mania to depression.

Bipolar I is the classic manic-depressive illness, with fully developed manic episodes and episodes of severe depression. It is also
characterized by long periods of "hibernation," during which the
symptoms temporarily disappear (table 2.2). The number of episodes varies enormously, but people who have only one or two

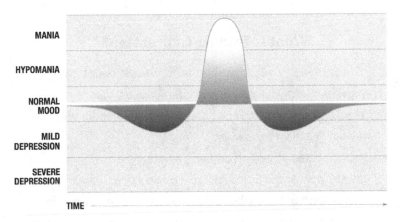

Figure 2.2. A triphasic mood episode, showing a period of depression followed by a period of mania and then another period of depression. It is not uncommon for psychiatrists to see patients who first sought treatment for the initial depressive phase and were put on an antidepressant, which triggered the patient's often-severe first manic episode. *Source: Illustration by Jenna Macfarlane.*

Table 2.2. Features of bipolar I

Mood

Fully developed manic episodes
Fully developed depressive episodes

Other features

Untreated episodes average six months
Hallucinations and delusions frequently seen
Three-phased episodes (depression, mania, depression)
Relapses more frequent as person ages

episodes seem to be the exception rather than the rule. Before effective treatments became available, the average length of each episode, if untreated, was about six months—but episodes that lasted years were not at all uncommon.

What Is "Manic-Depression"?

You may have come across the terms *manic-depression*, *manic-depressive illness* or *disorder*, or even *manic-depressive psychosis*. These are all older names for what we now call *bipolar disorder*.

In the late nineteenth century, a young German psychiatrist named Emil Kraepelin coined this term in the sixth edition of his textbook *Psychiatrie: Ein Lehrbuch* and applied it to all psychiatric illnesses characterized by recurrent episodes of abnormal mood—including cases that we would today call *major depressive disorder*. (I'll be quoting Dr. Kraepelin often in this book, as his observations and descriptions of people with bipolar disorder have stood the test of time.)

Manic-depression fell out of favor in the 1970s as it became clear that many people with this illness never develop full-blown manic states, but they nevertheless have both depressed mood episodes and other abnormal mood states at the opposite "pole" of the mood scale—thus, the term *bipolar* disorder.

Many people with bipolar I disorder experience nearly complete remission of their symptoms between episodes. This illness pattern often predicts that an individual will have an excellent response to treatment with lithium. Researchers at the University of Michigan studied the illness course of 209 cases of bipolar I disorder and found that about half of the subjects saw complete symptom remission between episodes. These people were completely free of symptoms almost ninety percent of the time. They called this the "stable" type of bipolar I disorder.

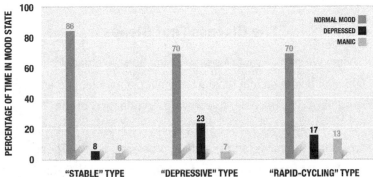

Figure 2.3. Three "data-driven" subtypes of bipolar I disorder. The height of the columns indicates the proportion of time that people spent in each mood state. In each subtype, individuals spent more time in a depressed state than in a manic state. *Source: Illustration by Jenna Macfarlane.*

The rest of the subjects fell somewhat evenly into two groups. One was a "depressed" group with at least some symptoms of depression twenty-three percent of the time. The other group was also symptom-free seventy percent of the time. Their symptomatic time was more or less evenly divided between depressive and manic symptoms. This last group, called "rapid-cycling," consisted of patients with briefer symptomatic periods that occurred more often. As mentioned above, the "stable" group has been recognized for years and is known to be more responsive to lithium. Being able to subdivide people who are less responsive to lithium into meaningful categories will hopefully lead to better ways to treat them (figure 2.3).

Bipolar II Disorder

People with *bipolar II disorder* have fully developed depressive episodes and episodes of hypomania. These people never develop full-blown mania, although they often have mild mixed states. A schematic representation of the moods of bipolar II appears in figure 2.4. The World Health Organization estimates that the lifetime prevalence of bipolar II disorder is 0.4 percent; about four in one thousand people develop the illness.

The Disease That Sleeps

When we think about illnesses of the body, we usually
think of diseases that have a beginning, a middle, and an
end. Take, for example, pneumonia, an infection of the
lungs caused by bacteria. The disease begins when fever,
cough, chest pains, and breathing problems appear. These
symptoms worsen over hours or sometimes days. Before
the antibiotic era, people reached a so-called *crisis* point,
when their bodies' natural defenses had mounted their best
effort against the bacterial invaders and the person either
started getting better or died. Either the person killed off the
bacteria or vice versa, but in any case the disease process
came to an end. (Fortunately, we can now administer
antibiotics that give the patient's defenses the crucial edge
against the bacterial invader.)

Bipolar disorder is very different from pneumonia because
it does not simply have a beginning, a middle, and an end.
Or perhaps it is more accurate to say that the illness seems
to have many beginnings and many endings. The symptoms
of bipolar disorder can develop in an individual and then,
without any treatment at all, the symptoms may go away for
years at a time.

Since most people are more familiar with diseases that
end when their symptoms go away, this is often very difficult
for people and their families to understand. The symptoms
of bipolar disorder can go into *remission* after treatment (or,
sometimes, even spontaneously). However, they almost

inevitably will come back if treatment to prevent their return is not in place. The hallmark of bipolar illness—especially bipolar I—is the tendency to *relapse*. Treatment can result in the complete remission of symptoms. They can disappear entirely. However, the illness does not end there. Instead, it seems merely to hibernate—and *symptoms can come back at any time*.

Initially, some researchers suspected that individuals with a history of hypomania and depression but not mania were in the early stages of "manic-depression." But several observational studies in the 1970s and '80s showed that this was not the case. One of these, written by Dr. William Coryell and his colleagues, followed people with recurrent depressions and hypomania for some years and found that fewer than five percent of them ever became manic. Bipolar II is not merely a prelude to "full-blown" manic-depressive illness, and people with bipolar II are not in the early stages of bipolar I.

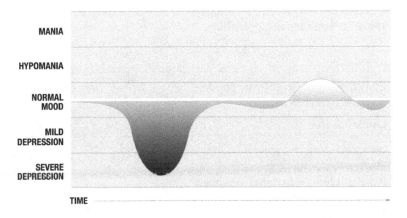

Figure 2.4. Mood changes in bipolar II. *Source: Illustration by Jenna Macfarlane.*

Bipolar II: What to Expect

Bipolar II is sometimes erroneously referred to as a milder form of bipolar I. Although people with bipolar II do not develop the most severe symptoms of full-blown mania, they tend to have symptoms more of the time. Long periods of depression are typical of bipolar II disorder and can be even more debilitating than the dramatic but shorter-lived episodes of bipolar I illness (table 2.3).

A 2011 study out of South Korea, titled "Differences between Bipolar I and Bipolar II Disorders in Clinical Features," outlined the many differences between symptom patterns in the two illnesses. These researchers found that people with bipolar II are more likely to have a seasonal variation in their symptoms. "Seasonal variation" means that they tend to get depressed in the fall and winter and feel better—or even develop hypomania—in the spring and summer. Also, they tend to have more rapid cycling. Whereas individuals with bipolar I frequently have irritable manic symptoms, the hypomanic periods of individuals with bipolar II are characterized by an elated mood. Irritability is less common.

With regard to depressive symptoms, people with bipolar II disorder more often suffer from psychomotor agitation (unintentional movements with no purpose, such as pacing, rapid talking,

Table 2.3. Features of bipolar II

Mood

Fully developed depressive episodes
Hypomanic episodes

Other features

Increased sleep and appetite during depressions
Depressions sometimes more chronic
Bipolar II history in family members
Later age at first hospitalization
Fewer hospitalizations
Possible increased risk for alcoholism

or tapping one's fingers or toes), guilty feelings, and thoughts of suicide. People with bipolar II also have a higher incidence of phobias and eating disorders. Typically, hypomanic episodes taper off as the person with bipolar II ages. When they reach middle age, depression is usually the predominant mood.

Cyclothymic Disorder

People with *cyclothymic disorder* have short, frequent periods of depressive symptoms and hypomania, separated by brief periods of normal mood. By definition, the person does not have either fully developed major depressive episodes or fully developed manic episodes. A schematic representation of the moods of cyclothymia appears in figure 2.5. These individuals essentially cycle almost continuously between mild depression and mild elation.

Emil Kraepelin, the German psychiatrist who developed the modern concept of bipolar illnesses, reported that three to four percent of his patients had cyclothymia. He speculated that many more people might have similar illnesses that "run their course outside of institutions." For many years, American psychiatric classification systems considered cyclothymia an expression of a person's personality rather than an illness caused by abnormal

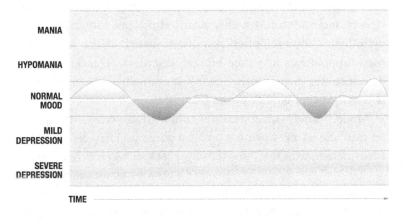

Figure 2.5. Mood changes in cyclothymia. *Source: Illustration by Jenna Macfarlane.*

brain chemistry. In early editions of the *Diagnostic and Statistical Manual of Mental Disorders* of the American Psychiatric Association (the *DSM*), the disorder was called *cyclothymic personality disorder*. In 1980, *cyclothymic disorder* moved over to the mood-disorder section of the manual—where it remains today.

Table 2.4. Features of cyclothymic disorder

Mood
Frequent alternation between mild depression and mild hypomania
Short, irregular cycles (days)
Only short periods of normal mood

Other features
People often wake up with mood changes
Pattern appears in late teens, early twenties
Frequently mistaken for problem with "personality"
Sometimes develops into bipolar I or II

Cyclothymia is now considered a subtype of bipolar disorder, a classification supported by family-history studies. People with cyclothymia often have relatives with bipolar disorder but rarely have relatives suffering from depression only. Treatment experiences seem to confirm this relationship: the mood swings of cyclothymic disorder often respond to many of the same treatment approaches as other bipolar disorders. This finding also demonstrates that cyclothymia is just as much a "chemical" problem as the other bipolar disorders.

Modern studies on community populations have come up with an estimate of between 0.4 and 2.4 percent. They estimate that many people with the disorder never seek or receive treatment.

Cyclothymic Disorder: What to Expect
Individuals with cyclothymic disorder have frequent ups and downs of mood, with only comparatively few periods of "normal" mood, as seen in table 2.4. (This almost constant instability per-

haps explains why psychiatrists thought of this as a "personality" characteristic for so long.) As might be expected, constant mood instability causes instability in many areas of the person's life. In a 1979 study of forty-six patients with cyclothymia, the patients demonstrated various oscillations of emotions and behavior— from sleep patterns to work habits to group affiliations—which can be seen in table 2.5.

Table 2.5. Mood, thinking, and behavior patterns in forty-six cyclothymic patients

Mood	Percentage of patients
Irritable periods lasting a few days	50
Explosive, aggressive outbursts	50
Thinking	
Shaky self-esteem alternating between lack of self-confidence and overconfidence	75
Periods of mental confusion alternating with periods of sharpened, creative thinking	50
Activity and behavior	
Increased sleep alternating with decreased need for sleep	75
Unevenness in quantity and quality of work	75
Buying sprees, extravagance, or financial disasters	75
Repeated shifts in work, study, interest, or future plans	50
Drug or alcohol abuse	50
Extroversion alternating with introversion	50
Unexplained promiscuity or extramarital affairs	40
Joining new movement with enthusiasm, rapidly changing to disillusionment	25

Source: Data from H. S. Akiskal, M. K. Khani, and A. Scott-Strauss, "Cyclothymic Temperamental Disorders," *Psychiatric Clinics of North America* 2, no. 3 (1979): 527–54; quoted in Frederick K. Goodwin and Kay Redfield Jamison, *Manic-Depressive Illness* (New York: Oxford University Press, 1990), 54.

Cyclothymic disorder tends to begin very early in life. A study of 894 young patients (aged 5 to 17 years old) found that nearly three-quarters of the patients with cyclothymic disorder had first experienced symptoms before they were 10 years old. As a group, they had a younger onset of illness than people with clinical depression or bipolar II disorder.

Many people with cyclothymic disorder never develop more severe mood symptoms. However, studies have shown that a significant number eventually develop a manic episode or severe depression—that is, they turn out to have bipolar I or II. However, perhaps half of all individuals with the cyclothymic pattern never develop symptoms of full-blown bipolar disorder. This finding shows that cyclothymic disorder is a valid condition in its own right.

"Soft" Bipolar Disorders

"Soft" bipolar disorders are mood disorders that have some features of bipolar disorder but don't fit the pattern of better-defined subtypes (table 2.6). Psychiatrists have long recognized that there are many forms of bipolar disorder. Emil Kraepelin noted that "it is fundamentally and practically impossible to keep apart in any way" the various forms of bipolar disorder. He stated, "Everywhere there are transitions."

Clinicians often see patients who come to them for symptoms of depression and have an illness that seems related to bipolar

Table 2.6. Indicators of "soft" bipolar disorders

Indicators
Family history of bipolar disorder
History of mania or hypomania caused by treatment with antidepressants
History of "mixed" mood states
Depressive, "hyper," or cycling temperament
Recurrent depressions

Depression—or Bipolar Disorder?

In the 1970s, the National Institutes of Health began a study on 559 people diagnosed with a depressive disorder. One of the aims of the study was to see how a serious depressive illness evolved in individuals over their lifetimes. The researchers followed some of these volunteers for up to thirty-one years.

In 1995, researchers published a series of reports with results from the first ten or so years of the study. One of those papers reported that nearly nine percent of these individuals with "depression" developed a hypomanic episode during that time; that is, they turned out to have bipolar II disorder.* The first hypomanic episode usually occurred within several months of the onset of depression, but sometimes it took up to nine years for the correct diagnosis to become apparent. Occasionally, these people with "depression" developed a manic episode—that is, they turned out to have bipolar I—but this was far less common (only 3.9 percent).

People with depression who later developed hypomanic periods (the people with bipolar II disorder) were about five years younger when they first developed depression. Their first episodes of depression were significantly longer—nearly three times as long.

*H. S. Akiskal, J. D. Maser, P. J. Zeller, J. Endicott, W. Coryell, M. Keller, M. Warshaw, P. Clayton, and F. Goodwin, "Switching from 'Unipolar' to Bipolar II: An 11-Year Prospective Study of Clinical and Temperamental Predictors in 559 Patients," *Archives of General Psychiatry* 52, no. 2 (1995): 114–23. https://doi.org/10.1001/archpsyc.1995.03950140032004.

In 2011, another report on these same individuals was published. It was now thirty-one years since the bout of depression that initially brought them into the study. With the passage of more time, nearly one in five of the people with "depression" had developed some form of bipolar disorder (19.6 percent); 12.2 percent had developed bipolar II, and 7.5 percent had developed bipolar I.*

This report also noted that subjects who reported even a few hypomanic symptoms at the beginning of the study were at greater risk of developing bipolar disorder. Also, the more symptoms they reported, the higher their risk was of developing bipolar disorder.

These studies found that people with "depression" who go on to develop a bipolar disorder (either bipolar I or II) were

- younger when they first developed a major depression,

- more likely to have a relative with a diagnosis of bipolar disorder, and

- more likely to have a few mild hypomanic symptoms.

*J. G. Fiedorowicz, J. Endicott, A. C. Leon, D. A. Solomon, M. B. Keller, and W. H. Coryell, "Subthreshold Hypomanic Symptoms in Progression from Unipolar Major Depression to Bipolar Disorder," *American Journal of Psychiatry* 168, no. 1 (2011): 40–48. https://doi.org/10.1176/appi.ajp.2010.10030328.

disorder. Terms like *pseudo-unipolar depression* and *bipolar III* describe various types of severe depressions with some features of bipolar disorder that do not fall into traditional categories for bipolar diagnoses. Currently, none of these terms have found their way into official diagnostic systems like the *DSM*.

As more treatments for bipolar disorder become available and more research on mood disorders is done, it is becoming clear that many people who suffer from mainly depressive symptoms can benefit from treatment with medications for bipolar disorders.

For about a half-century, psychiatry divided mood disorders into cases of unipolar depression, an illness characterized by only depressive symptoms, and bipolar disorders, in which people suffer depressive episodes but also manic, hypomanic, or mixed states.

"Soft" bipolar disorders seem to challenge this way of thinking; many of these people have an illness dominated by depressive symptoms with only the slightest colorings of mania. Sometimes, a family history of bipolar disorder is the only hint. More frequently, they have brief periods of elevated mood that they don't feel are particularly abnormal but that, when examined more closely, bear the hallmarks of hypomania: the decreased need for sleep, increased energy, uncharacteristic overconfidence, and loss of inhibitions. They can have periods of agitation and irritability that last only a few hours and possibly represent mild mixed states.

I have seen many patients who have taken one antidepressant after another for what they have been told is "unipolar depression," to little or no avail. For many of these patients, there are bipolar features in their illness that haven't been recognized as such. When these patients take a medication more typically used to treat bipolar disorder, their depressive symptoms frequently— and significantly—improve.

The Mood Disorder Spectrum

Emil Kraepelin, who coined the term *manic depressive disorder*, argued that all people with mood disorders should be diagnosed with "manic-depression." That would also include people who only have symptoms of depression. This idea fell out of favor in the first half of the twentieth century. That is when the term *unipolar depression* was coined, and psychiatrists started classifying purely depressive illnesses separately from bipolar disorders.

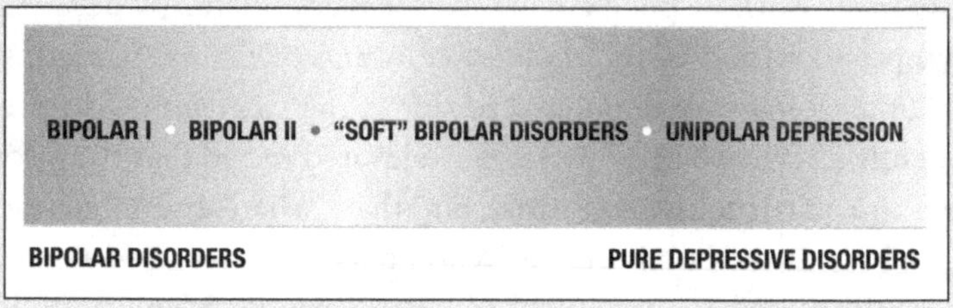

BIPOLAR I • BIPOLAR II • "SOFT" BIPOLAR DISORDERS • UNIPOLAR DEPRESSION

BIPOLAR DISORDERS   PURE DEPRESSIVE DISORDERS

Figure 2.6. The "spectrum" of mood disorders, from pure "unipolar" depression to bipolar I. *Source: Illustration by Jenna Macfarlane.*

Today, many mood disorder researchers argue that Kraepelin was right. They suggest that mood disorders vary along a *spectrum*, with pure depressive disorders at one end, bipolar I disorder at the other, and many individuals in between.

A review paper published in 2007 found more than eleven hundred articles that argue either for or against this idea.* I would argue that most psychiatrists who treat patients with mood disorders eventually come to agree with Dr. Kraepelin—they see patients every day who don't fit neatly into a *DSM* category.

* F. Benazzi, "Is There a Continuity between Bipolar and Depressive Disorders?," *Psychotherapy and Psychosomatics* 76, no. 2 (2007): 70–76. https://doi.org/10.1159/000097965.

Key Takeaways

❖ *Bipolar disorder is classified according to the mood states that are present during the patient's illness. Bipolar I, bipolar II, and cyclothymic disorder are well-defined. There is disagreement about how to classify the many other variations of the illness that can occur, the so-called "soft" bipolar disorders.*

❖ *There is at present no blood test or brain scan that can diagnose bipolar disorder. Psychiatrists make a diagnosis by gathering information from the patient about family history and the types and patterns of symptoms.*

PART II

How Is Bipolar Disorder Treated?

❖The successful treatment of bipolar disorder has three components:

- *Medication*
- *Psychotherapy and counseling*
- *Mood hygiene* (a collection of lifestyle changes that contribute to better control of symptoms)

Although there is at present no cure for bipolar disorder, there are many effective treatments that can control its symptoms for the majority of those who have it. In this and the following two chapters, I will survey these treatments one by one.

Like many other human diseases, mood disorders must be managed over time. Although there are no cures for high blood pressure or diabetes, there are practical approaches to addressing these problems and avoiding their complications: problems like heart attack, stroke, vision loss, and kidney failure. Those catastrophic problems can be prevented with good management of the underlying disorder. This management must continue throughout the person's lifetime. Bipolar disorder is no different. Its "complications" are just as dire: ruined relationships, wrecked finances, and, worst of all, suicide. And just as high blood pressure and diabetes can be effectively managed, so can bipolar disorder; its complications can be circumvented.

I can't emphasize strongly enough that each of these three components is crucial for the effective control of this illness. The best way to treat bipolar disorder is with these three very different but complementary treatment approaches. Leave out any one, and you'll soon find yourself tipping over into an episode of illness. Again, this is not so different from the approach to managing diabetes. Medication to keep blood sugar under control is essential, but learning about and implementing sound nutritional habits can't be neglected.

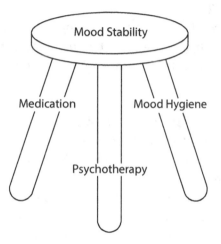

Figure II.1. Three components of treating bipolar disorder.

❖Because bipolar disorder is caused by problems with the brain's biological functioning, medications and other medical treatments to restore normal biological functioning are a crucial element of treatment.
Unhealthy neurons (the cells that are the fundamental units of the brain and nervous system) are believed to be a root cause of bipolar disorder. The medications that are effective in treating the illness work either by protecting neurons

or increasing their numbers in areas of the brain that are
important for emotional regulation. In chapters 3 through 6,
I will discuss these treatments in detail.

❖Bipolar disorder takes a psychological toll
on those who have it, and on their families
as well. Managing psychological stress is a
critical component of keeping symptoms from
returning.
Counseling and psychotherapy give a person with bipolar
disorder the psychological tools to better navigate a life that
this unforgiving illness has intruded into. Individual and group
therapy and support and educational groups have all been
shown to help prevent relapses and keep people with bipolar
disorder well. I'll review this component in chapter 7.

❖Bipolar disorder is a "stress-sensitive" disease.
Lifestyle changes that reduce psychological and
physical stress are a vital aspect of staying well.
This is such an important topic that I devoted a whole
section of the book to it and will discuss this topic at length
in part III.

CHAPTER 3

Mood-Stabilizing Medications

The foundation of medical treatment for bipolar disorder is a *mood-stabilizing medication*. These medications treat both depressive and manic symptoms and prevent mood episodes from recurring, an effect referred to as *prophylaxis* or *maintenance treatment*.

Lithium

Australian psychiatrist John Frederick Joseph Cade accidentally discovered the therapeutic effect of lithium for bipolar disorder in the late 1940s. While working in a large public psychiatric hospital in Melbourne, Cade became interested in measuring nitrogen-containing compounds in the urine of people with bipolar disorder. He tried injecting these compounds into guinea pigs to assess their effects on the animals' behavior, using lithium to make the compounds easier to dissolve. Cade soon realized that lithium was sedating the animals and thought it was perhaps a new sedative drug. He administered small doses of lithium to several psychiatric patients, and he observed a remarkable antimanic effect in people with bipolar disorder.

In the decade that followed Cade's discovery, the Danish psychiatrist Mogens Schou started administering lithium to people with bipolar disorder. He discovered that in addition to its antimanic and antidepressant effects, it helped prevent people from having relapses of their illness. In ensuing years, thousands more research articles on lithium appeared, making it perhaps the most studied drug in psychiatry. By the 1970s, lithium had become the standard by which all other treatments for bipolar disorder are judged, a position it holds to this day (table 3.1).

In the introduction to part II, I mentioned that many medications that are effective for bipolar disorder have a protective effect on neurons. Lithium is one of these and is thought to help through a *neuroprotective effect*. This lithium effect is so significant that imaging studies show actual increases in brain volume in people with bipolar disorder who respond to it. As might be expected, then, lithium's therapeutic effect has a slow onset. In early studies, lithium took weeks to start helping people with severe depression or mania. For this reason, severely ill individuals are usually prescribed other medications to take along with lithium, at least initially—medications that I will discuss in the next chapter.

Lithium's Therapeutic Profile
Lithium is a naturally occurring element found in mineral springs, seawater, and certain ores. Therapeutic lithium preparations usually contain lithium carbonate. When the carbonate ion is combined with sodium, it forms sodium carbonate (also known as ordinary baking soda).

Because it is an element, lithium is not metabolized, or chemically transformed, within the body. Since it is so similar to sodium, the body handles lithium in much the same way it handles sodium (salt). Lithium is rapidly absorbed through the gastrointestinal tract, enters the bloodstream, and is filtered through the kidneys and eliminated from the body. When a person starts taking lithium, it will take about five days for the level of medication to stabilize in the body. This means that if the lithium dose is changed, it will take about five days for the blood level to stabilize at the new level.

Lithium has a low *therapeutic index*, meaning that the difference between a therapeutic dose and a toxic dose is small. Fortunately, lithium can be measured in the bloodstream accurately and

Table 3.1. Therapeutic profile of lithium

Medication class	Mood stabilizer
Brand names	Eskalith, Eskalith-CR, Lithobid, Lithonate, Lithotabs
Half-life	14–30 hours
Metabolism	None
Elimination	Kidneys
Other considerations	Blood levels extremely important

cheaply, and the dosage can be adjusted according to the results.

It is important to pay attention to lithium blood levels not only to prevent toxicity but also because it has been demonstrated in clinical studies that lithium needs to be present in the bloodstream at a certain level to be effective in most people. (We speak of a "therapeutic level" in discussing the effective range of lithium in the bloodstream for treatment, not a "normal level." Lithium is a trace element in the body, usually present in undetectable concentrations.) Experts disagree on the optimal lithium level to treat bipolar disorder, but levels of 0.5 to 0.8 milliequivalents per liter (mEq/L) are considered standard. Some people have good control of their symptoms on even lower levels—elderly people, for example. Lithium levels thus need to be individualized to the patient. Dr. Schou, who might be thought of as the father of lithium therapy, pointed out that "changes in lithium levels as small as 0.1 to 0.2 [mEq/L], upward or downward, may substantially improve patients' quality of life during maintenance treatment."

Lithium levels (and the levels of most other drugs, for that matter) need to be measured twelve hours after the patient's last dose. The most convenient way to accomplish this is to arrive at the lab for blood work twelve hours after the bedtime dose. For example, if the bedtime dose was taken at eleven p.m. the night before, the person should arrive by eleven a.m. the next morning—with their usual morning dose in their pocket or purse.

For some people with bipolar disorder, lithium is uniquely effective. For them, it is necessary and sufficient, truly a miracle drug. In many of these people, other medications simply don't control their symptoms as well.

Lithium's Side Effects

Many medication side effects are *dose-related*, meaning that the higher the dose is, the more severe the side effect will be. Lithium is no exception. This is why physicians will try to maintain their patients at the lowest dose that controls their symptoms.

Because of its similarity to sodium, lithium has some of the

Symptoms of Lithium Toxicity

The difference between a therapeutic blood level and a toxic blood level of lithium is significantly smaller than with most other drugs. This fact makes it essential for people taking lithium to become familiar with the symptoms of too much lithium in the bloodstream, or *lithium toxicity*. Older people are especially vulnerable to lithium toxicity. It's helpful to divide the kinds of lithium toxicity into two types, shown below.

Acute toxicity occurs when a person's lithium level is *suddenly* too high. This can happen when a person mistakenly takes an extra dose of lithium, if they are significantly dehydrated, or as a result of intentional overdose. The symptoms are mainly in the digestive tract:

- Diarrhea

- Nausea and vomiting

- Stomach pains

- Dizziness

- Muscle weakness

Chronic toxicity occurs when the lithium level has slowly risen over a long time to toxic levels. This can happen in a person whose dose has changed or in whom kidney problems are developing. Digestive symptoms are less common, and nervous system issues predominate:

- Slowed thinking or confusion

- Severe tremor (shaking, usually most noticeably in the hands)

- Slurred speech

- Unsteady walk or problems with balance

In either type of toxicity, excessively high lithium levels can lead to coma or even death. Significant signs of lithium toxicity represent a medical emergency worth a trip to the emergency room for treatment.

same effects that increased sodium (salt) intake would have: increased thirst and urination and water retention. These side effects are often temporary and subside as the body adjusts to the medication. Lithium's side effects are summarized in table 3.2.

Lithium is irritating to the gastrointestinal tract and can cause nausea or diarrhea. Taking it on a full stomach can ease these problems considerably. A fine shaking in the hands (tremor) can occur at higher dosage levels. Slow-release preparations, which reduce the peak blood level that occurs after each dose, can alleviate these symptoms. Medications used to treat tremors, called *beta-blockers*, are frequently prescribed and can be very helpful.

Weight gain can be an annoying side effect and, unfortunately, has an equally annoying remedy: diet and exercise.

Between five and thirty-five percent of people treated with lithium develop depressed thyroid gland functioning (hypothyroidism). This may cause an increase in mood cycling in addition to

Lithium's Robust "Anti-suicide" Effect

People with bipolar disorder are at high risk of suicide; their suicide rate is twenty to thirty times higher than that of the general population. Half of those with an early age of onset have a history of suicide attempts. Fortunately, in addition to its ability to prevent illness episodes, lithium has a specific "anti-suicide" effect.

Many research studies have shown that lithium has a significant effect on reducing suicide attempts and deaths by suicide compared with antidepressants or other mood stabilizers in people with bipolar disorder. Long-term treatment with lithium reduces suicide attempts by about ten percent and deaths by suicide by about twenty percent.

A 2016 review of these studies in the French psychiatry journal *L'Encéphale* concluded that it is "crucial for . . . suicide prevention" to maintain lithium blood levels in the therapeutic range over the long term.* Lithium has a modulating effect on serotonin circuits in the brain that are involved with impulsiveness and aggressiveness. These are the vulnerability factors that put people with bipolar disorder at a higher risk of suicide.

*V. Benard, G. Vaiva, M. Masson, and P. A. Geoffroy, "Lithium and Suicide Prevention in Bipolar Disorder," *L'Encéphale* 42, no. 3 (2016): 234–41. https://doi.org/10.1016/j.encep.2016.02.006.

the symptoms of too little thyroid hormone (low energy, dry skin, sensitivity to heat, and puffiness around the eyes are some of the early signs). If a person's lithium seems to "stop working"—that is, if a person who is doing well suddenly seems to have an acceleration in their illness—hypothyroidism should be suspected. When it does occur, it can be treated by thyroid replacement medications. Blood tests of thyroid functioning are routinely ordered to monitor for this problem.

Lithium can cause flare-ups of preexisting skin conditions but only rarely causes new dermatological problems. People with psoriasis, acne, and other such problems may need to pay a follow-up visit to their dermatologist.

Another side effect that troubles a significant number of people taking lithium is a noticeable dulling of mental functioning and coordination. They complain that their ability to memorize and learn is affected and that they have a difficult-to-explain sense of mental sluggishness. This is a dose-related side effect and is another reason to strive for the lowest possible maintenance dose of lithium that still adequately controls mood symptoms.

Over the longer term, lithium can affect kidney functioning and cause an increase in urination. This problem develops slowly,

Table 3.2. Treatable side effects of lithium

Side effect	Remedy
Nausea, diarrhea	Take immediately after meals
	Switch preparations
Weight gain	Diet and exercise
Water retention	Diuretics helpful but must be prescribed by an MD
Tremor	Beta-blockers
Flare-up of preexisting dermatologic conditions	Dermatologic preparations
Hypothyroidism	Thyroid medications

is easy to diagnose with laboratory tests, and is treatable with ami-
loride. This drug changes how the kidneys reabsorb water and
other agents. When caught early on, this problem is usually completely reversible, so it's critical that people taking lithium let their
doctor know if they find themselves awakening more often to uri-
nate during the night.

When lithium was first prescribed, there were reports that
lithium disrupted the kidneys' filtering system and could cause
the kind of damage that can result in the need for dialysis. We
now know that this is extremely rare, occurring almost entirely in
people already at risk for kidney damage from other causes. These
include problems such as poorly controlled high blood pressure
or diabetes. Fortunately, this problem usually takes decades to
develop. Because of these potential problems, prescribers will
order blood tests that measure kidney function for people taking
lithium along with the blood test to monitor their lithium blood
levels.

Lithium can cause certain rare congenital heart defects, but
the risk is extremely low. What to do about taking lithium during
pregnancy is a complicated decision that should be discussed well
beforehand with your psychiatrist and your obstetrician. Lithium
is secreted in breast milk, so people taking lithium should not
breastfeed.

Key Takeaways about Lithium

❖ *Lithium continues to be the gold standard treatment for bipolar disorder, especially for people with bipolar I.*

❖ *Lithium is a "magic bullet" for many people with bipolar I: both necessary and sufficient to keep them well.*

❖ *Lithium blood tests are essential, but interpreting the results is best
left to an expert. The optimal level for an individual person depends on
factors such as illness phase, the severity of symptoms, and age.*

❖ *Women in their childbearing years taking lithium should have a pregnancy-planning discussion with their prescriber. Many women decide that the effects of an illness episode on the baby outweigh the very low risk of birth defects.*

Lamotrigine (Lamictal)

As is true of several other medications I will discuss in this chapter, the first use of lamotrigine was to treat seizure disorders. It was first used as an "add-on" drug for people with epilepsy who were already taking other antiseizure medications. Researchers noted that people who took lamotrigine for seizure control reported improved mood and sense of well-being—even if it hadn't helped much with their seizures. These observations led to clinical trials in people with mood disorders, which quickly revealed that lamotrigine is an effective medication for many such people.

Like lithium, lamotrigine appears to have neuroprotective effects that explain its effectiveness in treating bipolar disorder.

Lamotrigine's Therapeutic Profile

In 2003, two large studies were published comparing the efficacy of lamotrigine with lithium (and with a placebo) in keeping people with bipolar disorder from having another mood episode; each study lasted eighteen months. In one study, the individuals were recovering from a manic or mixed episode as they entered the study; in the other, they were recovering from depression. When both studies reported that lamotrigine was just as effective as lithium in keeping people with bipolar disorder well, this new medication suddenly came into the spotlight. It quickly became one of the foundations of the treatment of bipolar disorder.

The exciting finding from these studies was that lamotrigine is especially effective against depression in bipolar disorder—excellent news. This was such an important finding because, as you will see later, the depression in bipolar disorder is much more challenging to treat than manic or mixed states. You may remember from chapter 2 that individuals with bipolar II disorder have more problems with depression than with mania and that these depressions can be long, debilitating, and difficult to treat. Lamotrigine can often fill a critical therapeutic need for these people because lithium is often less effective for them (table 3.3). Conversely, lamotrigine appears to be less effective than lithium for people with bipolar I disorder.

Blood-level tests are not routinely ordered for lamotrigine because of its low toxicity and because therapeutic effects have not been correlated with particular amounts in the blood.

Lamotrigine's Side Effects

In contrast to other mood stabilizers, lamotrigine causes only minimal side effects. People taking it may have some initial nausea or gastrointestinal upset and the sort of side effects that many medications affecting the brain can cause—sleepiness, light-headedness or dizziness, and headaches. At higher doses, some people complain of concentration problems similar to those often reported by people taking lithium. In my experience, lowering the dose usually takes care of this problem.

A rare but serious problem that has been associated with lamotrigine is a dangerous type of allergic skin rash called *toxic epidermal necrolysis* (TED). TED is the most extreme form of a group of allergic skin reactions that are lumped together under the term *erythema multiforme*. These problems were reported right after lamotrigine was introduced as a treatment for epilepsy in the early 1990s. When research was done to see who was at the highest risk for these serious reactions, it was discovered that children and individuals who started the drug at high doses were more likely than others to develop a serious rash. Now, people start lamotrigine at a low dose (about one-tenth of the ultimate therapeutic dose) and gradually increase it over a period of weeks. Although this means that it may take five weeks or more to get to the usual therapeutic dose of 200 to 400 milligrams (mg)/day, the risk of serious skin reactions to lamotrigine has virtually been eliminated.

Remember that individuals can develop *minor* skin reactions to

Table 3.3. Therapeutic profile of lamotrigine

Medication class	Mood stabilizer (anticonvulsant)
Brand name	Lamictal
Half-life	5–24 hours
Metabolism	Affected by carbamazepine, valproate
Elimination	Liver
Other considerations	Rarely causes severe skin rashes but otherwise has good side-effect profile

medications, and lots of other things as well, so when a person starts taking lamotrigine, it's important for them to take precautions against developing a rash from another source. If a rash develops in a person taking lamotrigine, it presents something of a therapeutic dilemma: Is the person's rash erythema multiforme or a minor skin reaction? If the rash is a serious one, is lamotrigine the culprit? The person might be told to stop the drug unnecessarily, perhaps missing out on a medication that might be highly effective. For this reason, people starting on lamotrigine should consider the protocol developed at Stanford University to prevent skin rashes from other sources (table 3.4). I had one patient who had been told by her previous psychiatrist to stop lamotrigine, which up to that point had seemed very helpful for her bipolar depression, because she had developed what in retrospect was probably a reaction to poison ivy. She was able to restart lamotrigine and move up to a therapeutic dose with no problems. I tell my patients as I hand them the prescription, "No gardening, no hiking, no new restaurants, or shampoos or clothes detergents; stay out of the sun, and take care of your skin!"

I have seen people with bipolar disorder who have appeared to greatly benefit from taking lamotrigine but who developed mild erythema multiforme on it. Several studies have shown—and I have seen—that sometimes, by starting at a tiny dose and increasing the level more slowly than usual, people can safely get to a therapeutic dose and stay on it. Obviously, a careful risk-versus-benefit

Table 3.4. Stanford protocol for patients starting lamotrigine

Do not start lamotrigine within two weeks of any rash, viral
  infection, or vaccination.
Take precautions outdoors to prevent sunburn and contact with
  poison ivy, oak, or sumac.
During the first three months of treatment, avoid exposure as much
  as possible to any new
  • medicines
  • foods
  • soaps, cosmetics, conditioners, or deodorants
  • detergents or fabric softeners

discussion needs to occur before embarking on such a plan, and
very close monitoring is needed.

A corollary to the start-low protocol for lamotrigine is that a
person who stops taking it for a period of time should not resume
taking it at the same dose. Experts recommend that people who
are off lamotrigine for one week or more should restart the drug
at the low beginning dose.

Key Takeaways about Lamotrigine

❖ *Lamotrigine appears to be especially effective for bipolar depression in
people with bipolar II.*

❖ *The side-effect profile is excellent.*

❖ *The risk of serious dermatological reactions is real but quite low; following the Stanford protocol for avoiding rashes is well worth the effort.*

❖ *Even people who develop a rash can often have a "re-challenge" and
take lamotrigine.*

❖ *People taking lamotrigine who go without it for more than a week
should restart the induction process at a low dose.*

Carbamazepine (Tegretol, Equetro, Epitol)

After the introduction of carbamazepine for the control of epilepsy in the 1960s, several reports appeared indicating that people with epilepsy who took carbamazepine and also had mood problems not only developed good control over their seizures but saw improvement in their psychiatric symptoms as well. It was a small step to test carbamazepine in people with mood problems who did not have epilepsy.

Carbamazepine's Therapeutic Profile

Although carbamazepine has been used to treat bipolar disorder for several decades, less research has been done on its efficacy in treating this illness than for other medications. This gap is slowly being filled, however, and newer studies have appeared, prompted by the development of a sustained-release preparation.

Carbamazepine is used to treat bipolar disorder less often for three reasons. First, it doesn't seem to have any big advantage over other mood stabilizers in most studies of groups of individuals. Second, it is tricky to dose effectively. And third, there is a low risk of serious side effects.

Regarding the lack of advantage over other mood stabilizers, there is even one well-designed double-blind study that found that people with mania who took carbamazepine actually seemed to do *worse* than people taking lithium. Nevertheless, most psychiatrists (including this one) have had a patient like "Ms. B.," whose case history was reported in a paper from the National Institute of Mental Health (NIMH) in 1983:

> Ms. B., a 53-year-old woman, had a history of treatment-resistant, rapid-cycling manic-depressive illness that required continuous state hospitalization from 1956 to her admission to NIMH in 1978. She had been non-responsive to [antipsychotic medications, antidepressants] and lithium . . . After institution of carbamazepine, both mood phases improved dramatically and she was able to be discharged . . . During a

subsequent hospitalization, her severe mania again did not respond to [antipsychotic medications] and she was not able to leave the hospital until she was treated with carbamazepine.

Carbamazepine, although not a first or even second choice in mood stabilizers, is nevertheless a welcome addition to our arsenal of drugs for bipolar disorder, as it helps some people who have failed to benefit from other medications (table 3.5).

Carbamazepine's dosing issue is that it causes the liver to increase the level of the enzymes that metabolize it. This means that the longer a person takes carbamazepine, the more quickly the liver gets rid of it. So after a few weeks, the blood levels may go down and the dose may need to be increased. This increase in liver enzymes can also affect other medications that the person might be taking, including certain tranquilizers, antidepressants, hormones, and other epilepsy medications. The change in hormonal levels is very important for women using birth control, since some oral contraceptives that use low hormone levels lose their effectiveness if taken with carbamazepine. It is critical that all physicians involved in a person's care know when the person has started taking carbamazepine so that dosage adjustments for other medications can be made.

Table 3.5. Therapeutic profile of carbamazepine

Medication class	Mood stabilizer (anticonvulsant)
Brand names	Tegretol, Equetro, Epitol
Half-life	18–15 hours (shortens over time)
Metabolism	Complex; affects and is affected by other drugs
Elimination	Liver
Other considerations	Blood-level tests helpful; blood tests for liver inflammation and blood abnormalities needed

Carbamazepine's Side Effects

Carbamazepine can cause the same sort of general side effects as many other medications that affect the brain: sleepiness, light-headedness, and some initial nausea. These problems tend to be short-lived and dose-related.

There have been rare cases of liver problems associated with carbamazepine, so blood tests for liver inflammation are routinely done. There have been even rarer reports of dangerous changes in blood cell counts, so routine blood cell counts are also done, especially in the first several weeks of therapy. Cases of a dangerous skin reaction called Stevens-Johnson syndrome have been attributed to carbamazepine; this is another one of the severe variants of erythema multiforme that I mentioned in the discussion of lamotrigine. All these problems are quite rare, but are the third reason for this drug's relative lack of use. People taking carbamazepine should be on the lookout for the development of a rash, jaundice (yellowing of the eyes and skin), water retention, bleeding or bruising, or signs of infection.

Oxcarbazepine (Trileptal)

As its name suggests, oxcarbazepine (brand name Trileptal) is closely related to carbamazepine, but has several impressive advantages over the parent compound. It is not associated with the blood-cell count problems that can be caused by carbamazepine or with the changes in liver enzymes that affect the metabolism of other drugs. This makes it significantly easier to take, with less need for monitoring blood tests and changes in dosage. It also appears less likely to cause Stevens-Johnson syndrome. Much of the early work on oxcarbazepine in bipolar disorder was done in Europe, and studies by German investigators in the mid-1980s suggested it was as beneficial as carbamazepine in treating mania. More recently, many other research papers have been published that support its safety and efficacy, especially as an "add-on" to other mood stabilizers. The effectiveness of oxcarbazepine for

breakthrough manic symptoms has been especially well established, and reports of it being effective when taken alone have also
been published.

Many clinicians have been reluctant to prescribe oxcarbazepine's parent compound, carbamazepine, because of the possibility of severe adverse reactions. Given the fewer significant
problems associated with oxcarbazepine, we will probably see it
prescribed more often and studied more closely.

Key Takeaways about Carbamazepine/Oxcarbazepine

❖ *Both drugs have been shown to be effective in some people with bipolar
disorder, but neither have been studied as well as lithium or lamotrigine.*

❖ *Both drugs have been shown to help with breakthrough symptoms
when added to other medications.*

❖ *Published case reports support the efficacy of both these drugs taken
alone as a person's only mood stabilizer.*

❖ *Oxcarbazepine (Trileptal) may be as effective as carbamazepine
(Tegretol) in bipolar disorder, but with a lower risk of serious side effects.*

Valproate (Depakote, Depakene, Epival)

Valproic acid is a carbon compound similar to others that are
found in animal fats and vegetable oils; it is a fatty acid. It was first
synthesized in 1882 and was used for many years as an organic
solvent for a variety of purposes. Valproate was approved by the
US Food and Drug Administration for use in treating epilepsy in
1978. After the discovery that carbamazepine, also an anti-epileptic
medication, was effective in treating mania, interest in using
valproate in bipolar disorder grew. In the mid-1980s, American
psychiatrists conducted several studies on the use of valproate in
treating bipolar disorder, and ten years later valproate became a
frequently used medication for bipolar disorder.

As you will see, however, not only does valproate appear to be less effective than the drugs already discussed in this chapter (one can argue that it shouldn't even be called a "mood stabilizer"), but it also has a number of very serious side-effect problems.

Valproate's Therapeutic Profile

Valproate seems to have some advantages over lithium in the treatment of acute manic episodes. First, while lithium may take up to three weeks to have its full effect, valproate has been shown to start working within five days. Second, valproate also seems to be more effective for certain subgroups of people with mania: people with rapid cycling (four or more mood episodes per year) and people with mixed mania (a mixture of manic hyperactivity and pressured thinking with depressed or unpleasant mood). Third, valproate is much less toxic than lithium (table 3.6).

Controlled studies of the use of valproate to treat acute depression and to prevent recurrences of bipolar disorder have been less impressive. In fact, if one sticks to the more rigorous controlled studies, it can be argued that valproate should be used only to treat acute mania and that the lack of strong evidence for its benefit in combatting depression or for maintenance treatment argues against any other use in treating bipolar disorder. Nevertheless, as with carbamazepine, any psychiatrist with experience in treating people with mood disorders will tell you that some people need and benefit from valproate and that for them, it is extremely and

Table 3.6. Therapeutic profile of valproate

Medication class	Mood stabilizer (anticonvulsant)
Brand names	Depakene, Depakote, Epival
Half-life	6–16 hours
Metabolism	Affected by other anti-epilepsy drugs
Elimination	Liver
Other considerations	Blood-level tests helpful; blood tests for liver inflammation are needed

sometimes uniquely effective. It may be that these people have an unusual variant of bipolar disorder and that the benefit of valproate for these people gets lost in large studies, where they are vastly outnumbered by patients who do not respond to valproate.

Like lithium, valproate can be measured in the bloodstream. As with lithium, blood for a test of valproate levels should be drawn twelve hours after the last dose.

Valproate's Side Effects

Common side effects include stomach upset and sleepiness. These problems usually go away quickly. Increased appetite and weight gain are the most serious side effects. Mild tremor occurs as well and can be treated with beta-blockers. A few individuals report hair loss, usually temporary, which resolves even more quickly with the use of shampoos and vitamin preparations containing the minerals zinc and selenium.

Cases of severe liver problems have been reported in people taking valproate, but they have occurred almost exclusively in children taking the drug for control of epilepsy. Just to be on the safe side, however, people on valproate should have episodic blood tests to detect liver inflammation. Since valproate can also, in rare cases, lower the number of red and white blood cells, a complete blood count is usually done as well. These are rare problems, and when they do occur, they develop slowly and usually during the first six months of therapy. People on valproate should be on the lookout for signs of liver or blood-count problems, which include unusual bleeding and bruising, jaundice, fever, and water retention.

Valproate has been associated with the development of polycystic ovary syndrome in women. The symptoms of this syndrome are irregular menstrual periods, the development of facial hair and male-pattern hair loss, obesity, and ovarian cysts.

Valproate has been associated with birth defects, and women of childbearing age should practice birth control while taking valproate if there is any possibility of becoming pregnant.

Key Takeaways about Valproate

❖ *It's questionable whether valproate should be considered a "mood sta-bilizer," as it has only been clearly proven to be effective in treating acute mania. The evidence for prescribing it to treat bipolar depression and to prevent future episodes (prophylaxis) is weak.*

❖ *There is a substantial risk of weight gain, especially in women, in whom it can also cause significant gynecological and hormonal problems (polycystic ovary syndrome).*

Other Mood Stabilizers

Several other agents show promise for the treatment of bipolar disorder. For the most part, the potential of these medications is based on clinical trials in which the medication is added to the regimen of people already taking an established mood stabilizer such as lithium, but sometimes a few case reports of a therapeutic effect are enough to attract the attention of psychiatrists.

Pramipexole (Mirapex) is a medication that is usually used to treat Parkinson's disease and restless legs syndrome; it activates dopamine circuits in the brain. Several studies have shown prami-pexole to be an effective add-on treatment for bipolar depression not responding to mood stabilizers alone. As with other treatments that are especially helpful for bipolar depression, there is a risk of developing hypomanic or manic symptoms.

There is evidence that N-acetyl cysteine (NAC), an amino acid available as a nutritional supplement, may be useful as a mood stabilizer. A number of studies examining NAC as an add-on medication to other mood stabilizers have shown promising results, especially in bipolar depression. This discovery is especially exciting because the mechanism of action of NAC is different from that of any other mood stabilizer. NAC is a metabolic precursor to glu-tathione, a powerful antioxidant that occurs in brain tissue, suggesting that NAC, like other mood stabilizers, may work through neuroprotective mechanisms.

Tiagabine (Gabitril) and zonisamide (Zonegran) are other anti-epilepsy drugs that have attracted the interest of clinical researchers of bipolar disorder. Ongoing work may result in these drugs also being introduced as mood-stabilizing medications.

Key Takeaways

❖ *A medication is considered a "mood stabilizer" if it is effective in treating manic and depressive episodes and prevents future episodes from occurring.*

❖ *Lithium is arguably the gold standard for treatment of bipolar I disorder.*

❖ *Several medications originally developed to treat epilepsy have been repurposed to treat bipolar disorder and can be more effective than lithium for some people.*

CHAPTER 4

Atypical Antipsychotic and Antidepressant Medications

People often take antipsychotic and antidepressant medications along with their mood-stabilizing medications. Usually, this is to control residual or breakthrough symptoms. For some people, they will be temporary additions to mood stabilizers. Others will take them over the long term.

ATYPICAL ANTIPSYCHOTIC MEDICATIONS

The *atypicals*, developed in the 1990s from drugs initially used to treat schizophrenia, have potent effects on mood. This feature makes them some of the most frequently prescribed medications to treat bipolar disorder.

This group of medications has a rather misleading name, "anti-*psychotic*"—misleading because they are frequently used to treat problems other than psychosis. I would even argue that more people take them for mood disorders than for "psychotic" illnesses such as schizophrenia.

Psychosis is a mental state or disorder that severely impairs the affected person's ability to comprehend their environment and react to it appropriately. The layperson's definition of *psychotic* might be "out of touch with reality." Someone who hears voices (auditory hallucinations) or who has bizarre beliefs (delusions) is psychotic. The word also connotes severe disorganization of thinking and behavior, usually with restlessness and agitation. The full-blown manic syndrome is an excellent example of a state of psychosis, and we have already talked about "psychotic features" in depression. These medications are the mainstays of treatment for schizophrenia, a psychiatric illness in which hallucinations and delusions are the main symptoms and mood is relatively unaffect-

Thorazine and Beyond

In the 1930s, a group of pharmaceutical compounds with antihistamine and sedative properties was synthesized in Europe. One in particular, chlorpromazine (Thorazine), was found to be useful in surgical anesthesia because it deepened anesthetic sedation more safely than other available agents. In the early 1950s, two French psychiatrists carried out several clinical trials using chlorpromazine to treat highly agitated patients suffering from schizophrenia and mania. They hoped the drug would provide sedation for these profoundly ill patients, which it did—but these astute clinicians noticed that the medication did much more.

In addition to its quieting and sleep-promoting effects, chlorpromazine made the hallucinations and bizarre delusional beliefs of many people with schizophrenia practically disappear. It also decreased the severity of disorganized thinking and agitation seen in people with acute mania. Chlorpromazine, in other words, had a *specific* effect on the cluster of symptoms often referred to as "psychotic" symptoms. Thus the name for this group came about: *antipsychotic medications*.

ed. As you might expect, then, atypicals are quite effective for psychotic symptoms in those people with bipolar disorder who develop them. However, they have additional and significant antimanic and antidepressant effects that make them exceptionally helpful for the many people with mood disorders who never do.

More Than "Antipsychotic"

As we saw in part I of this book, episodes of bipolar disorder can sometimes include extremely frightening mental symptoms and dangerously disturbed behaviors. This is true of both depressed and manic episodes. And, as we saw in the previous chapter, mood stabilizers sometimes take weeks to begin working. What can help slow down the racing, pressured thoughts and bursting overactivity of the individual with mania before lithium starts working? This is where antipsychotic medications are helpful. Because their calming effects begin almost immediately, these medications are especially useful in acute mania. They are frequently part of the treatment for the severely ill person with mania. In cases of depression where the individual is highly restless and agitated, they can have similar beneficial effects.

Unlike their predecessors, the newer antipsychotic medications have potent effects on brain circuits that use a brain chemical that you've likely heard of: *serotonin*. Serotonin circuits appear to be very important in mood regulation. The label *atypical antipsychotic medications* (you may also see them referred to as *second-generation antipsychotics*) differentiates them from the older antipsychotic medicines that have only minimal effects on the serotonin system in the brain (table 4.1). The original antipsychotic medications are now often referred to as *typical antipsychotics*. They are rarely used nowadays to treat mood disorders. They are usually reserved to treat severe mania with agitation. Even then, they are not prescribed for very long. The main reasons for this are the side effects that they cause.

How Is the Brain like a House?

You have probably read about comparisons between the human brain and a computer, but in a rather interesting way, the brain is also like a house.

If your house is like mine, behind its walls are a number of circuits. The network of wiring that brings electricity into every room is the most obvious, but there are others as well. There's a network of piping that supplies water to the bathrooms and the kitchen. The HVAC system has a network of ducts circulating warm air in the winter and cool air in the summer. All these networks work together to make your house a comfortable environment in which to live.

Like your house, the brain has different circuits that work together to control bodily functions and mental experiences. Of course, the brain's circuitry is tremendously more complex than anything in your house. It has many, many more circuits, and there are complicated connections between different circuits. Each brain circuit uses a different chemical messenger to send its messages.

These chemical messengers are called *neurotransmitters*. You may have heard of one of them, *serotonin*, which is especially important in mood circuitry. Other neurotransmitters are probably just as important: *norepinephrine* and *dopamine* are two, and there are many more.

As you read through several following chapters, you will learn that many medications we use in psychiatry mainly work through their effects on neurotransmitters.

Table 4.1. Atypical antipsychotic medications

Pharmaceutical name	Brand name(s)
Aripiprazole	Abilify
Asenapine	Saphris
Brexpiprazole	Rexulti
Cariprazine	Vrayler
Clozapine	Clozaril
Lurasidone	Latuda
Olanzapine	Zyprexa, Zyprexa Zydis
Quetiapine	Seroquel
Risperidone	Risperdal
Sulpiride*	Dogmatil
Ziprasidone	Geodon

* Not approved for use or available in the United States.

Atypical Antipsychotic Medications' Therapeutic Profile

The first atypical antipsychotic, *clozapine*, was synthesized in the 1960s. However, it was not marketed in the United States until 1990.

Soon after psychiatrists started to prescribe clozapine, they found it highly effective for treating people with schizophrenia. This was true even for people who had derived little benefit from older antipsychotic medications. Dramatic case studies appeared of people with chronic treatment-resistant schizophrenia who basically "awakened" from years of unrelenting psychotic symptoms after they started clozapine. Cases like these sustained the interest of clinicians and pharmaceutical researchers in the drug. Before long, people with treatment-resistant mood disorders were treated with it as well.

A 1996 research article reported on the use of clozapine in twenty-five patients with acute mania. These were patients "for whom lithium, anticonvulsants and [traditional antipsychotics] had been ineffective" or had produced severe side effects. Almost three-quarters of the patients had "marked improvement" in their manic symptoms.

After the introduction of clozapine and the appearance of research papers describing its effectiveness for the treatment of mood disorders, drug developers got to work. Many more atypicals have now come along, and their introduction substantially expanded the number of treatment options for bipolar disorder.

It is now apparent that the atypical antipsychotic medications are helpful in all phases of bipolar disorder—mania *and* depression—as well as for ongoing treatment to prevent relapse (maintenance treatment). Although these drugs are somewhat effective as maintenance treatments when taken alone, prescribing an atypical as an "add-on" medication to a mood stabilizer such as lithium is significantly more effective. A 2016 study compared the effectiveness of taking an atypical alone versus an atypical plus a mood stabilizer in preventing relapse in people recovering from a manic episode. Over a period of one year, the individuals taking only an atypical relapsed four times more often than the individuals who also took a mood stabilizer.

The excellent news is that these medications have significant antidepressant effects in many people—another reason why calling them "antipsychotic" medications is inaccurate.

Practicing psychiatrists (including this one) will tell you that some of the atypicals seem to be more antimanic and others more antidepressant in their effect. Unfortunately, as of this writing, there is no research that might bear this out by comparing the results of different atypicals for mania and bipolar depression.

Atypical Antipsychotic Medications' Side Effects

The most significant side-effect problem with atypical antipsychotic medications is their tendency to make some individuals gain weight. Some atypicals are more likely than others to cause weight gain. Some atypicals are relatively "weight-neutral" and do not cause significant weight gain. Weight gain can cause people to develop such obesity-related problems as high cholesterol and even diabetes. One cause of the weight gain associated with some atypical antipsychotics is the stimulation of the brain's appetite center. However, recent research indicates that these medications probably affect several hormones that control how the body handles calories and stores fat. Blood tests for diabetes and high cholesterol are often done at the beginning of treatment and regularly after that in people taking antipsychotics for maintenance treatment. They are also routinely weighed. Everyone taking atypical antipsychotics should take steps to control possible weight gain by paying attention to their diet and getting regular exercise.

Atypicals and the Metabolic Syndrome

The term *metabolic syndrome* refers to a collection of factors that put a person at higher risk of developing problems such as heart attacks and stroke. These factors are

- Obesity

- Increased blood sugar levels (prediabetes or diabetes)

- Increased levels of cholesterol and triglycerides ("lipid" or fat molecules in the blood)

- Hypertension (high blood pressure)

There is evidence that the first of these factors, obesity, causes the other three in many people. Several atypicals cause significant increases in appetite that often lead to weight gain. However, some studies have shown that they cause disturbances in glucose metabolism independent of what is caused by weight gain.

People taking an atypical antipsychotic and their prescribers must stay on the lookout for the development of metabolic syndrome by tracking weight, testing for high blood sugar and lipid levels, and monitoring blood pressure. The American Diabetes Association also recommends annually measuring a person's waist circumference and noting any family history of diabetes.

Although several medications have been reported to reduce the risk of developing metabolic syndrome, the diabetes drug metformin (Glucophage) has the most consistently positive results. People taking metformin lose the most weight when they also make healthy lifestyle changes like adopting a healthier diet and exercising regularly.

P. Pramyothin and L. Khaodhiar, "Metabolic Syndrome with the Atypical Antipsychotics," *Current Opinion in Endocrinology, Diabetes and Obesity* 17, no. 5 (2010): 460–66. https://doi.org/10.1097/MED.0b013e32833de61c.

A rare but severe side effect of atypical antipsychotic medications is the development of problems with heart rhythm. These medications can change the heart's electrical activity, making it take longer for the heart muscle to "reset" electrically between heartbeats. This phenomenon is called *QT prolongation*. The letters *Q* and *T* refer to points on an electrocardiogram (ECG or EKG). QT prolongation is dangerous because it can lead to much more serious changes in the heart's electrical activities, such that the heartbeat becomes disorganized. One of these serious changes is called *torsades de pointes*, from its appearance on an EKG. This can cause a fainting spell, a stroke, or even sudden death. Fortunately, only a minority of people who develop QT prolongation go on to develop serious problems. Most of those who do have other underlying risk factors that can be identified and sometimes corrected.

Another issue with this group of drugs is their potential side effects on muscle function. This was a serious issue with their predecessors, the drugs now referred to as *typical antipsychotics*.

QT Prolongation and Risk Factors for Torsades de Pointes

■ Older than sixty-five years of age

■ Abnormally slow heart rate

■ Congenital (inherited) prolonged QT syndrome

■ Treatment with diuretics ("fluid pills")

■ Abnormally low blood levels of potassium, calcium, and/or magnesium

■ Female gender

■ Genetic predisposition

■ Preexisting heart disease, including a history of myocardial infarction (heart attack) or congestive heart failure

■ Advanced liver disease

■ Treatment with multiple drugs that also prolong the QT interval

Modified from M. Li and L. G. Ramos, "Drug-Induced QT Prolongation and Torsades de Pointes," *Pharmacy and Therapeutics* 42, no. 7 (2017): 473–77.

The search for drugs that didn't have this effect led to the development of the atypicals. Muscle stiffness, restlessness, and abnormal movements are some of the problems the medications in this category can cause.

The development of the atypicals was one of two dramatic advancements in treating mood disorders that occurred in the 1990s. The other was the development of the selective serotonin reuptake inhibitor (SSRI) antidepressants, starting with fluoxetine (Prozac). I would assert that the introduction of the atypicals was the more important of the two, as it arguably resulted in a new group of mood-stabilizing drugs. If a mood stabilizer doesn't completely control bipolar symptoms or an antidepressant doesn't completely control unipolar depression symptoms, one of the first interventions is usually to add an atypical. This makes them some of the most frequently prescribed medications in psychiatric practice.

Key Takeaways about Atypical Antipsychotics

❖ *Atypical antipsychotic medications offer both antimanic and antidepressant effects and are usually "add-on" medications to treat mood disorders.*

❖ *Some, though not all atypicals, cause increased appetite. This can lead to weight gain and even obesity. This weight gain puts the individual at higher risk of developing obesity-related problems, such as high blood pressure and type 2 diabetes.*

❖ *A rare but potentially life-threatening heart rhythm problem can affect some individuals who take these medications. People with a history of heart disease should be screened for risk factors and closely monitored while taking them.*

Movement and Muscle Tone Side Effects

The antipsychotic medications discussed in this chapter have the potential for adverse effects on muscle tone and movement. In textbook discussions of these medications, you will see these problems referred to as *extrapyramidal symptoms*, or EPS.

The term *extrapyramidal* contrasts this system with

another set of brain circuits called the *pyramidal system.*
(This name came about because the main fibers of this
system are carried in triangular bundles in the spinal cord
called the *spinal pyramids.*) The pyramidal system controls
the quick, accurate execution of fine muscle movement. The
extrapyramidal system makes sure that the rest of the body
moves as needed for the smooth and graceful execution of
these movements. Antipsychotic medications interfere with
this system and can cause various side effects that involve
the muscles and movement.

One of these is *pseudoparkinsonism.* You may know
that people who have Parkinson's disease have a slowed
and shuffling walk. They also seem to lose facial expression
because of stiffness in their facial muscles, and they often
have trembling of their hands. Pseudoparkinsonism consists
of these same symptoms.

Another possible side effect is an *acute dystonic reaction.*
This is a sudden muscular spasm, more common in young
males, usually involving the tongue and facial and neck
muscles. People taking antipsychotic medications can also
develop a distressing restlessness called *akathisia.* This is
felt mainly in the legs so that the individual feels the need to
walk or pace.

Fortunately, all these side effects are treatable, either by
lowering the dose of medication or adding one of several
medications used to treat Parkinson's disease. Although
uncomfortable, these side effects are not dangerous
and usually respond quickly to treatment once they are
encountered and identified.

Most of the typical antipsychotic medications can cause a side effect called *tardive dyskinesia*, or TD for short. In most people, it takes years for TD to develop. However, it occasionally develops after only weeks or months of taking an antipsychotic.

TD consists of repetitive, involuntary movements, usually of the facial muscles, often chewing, blinking, or lip-pursing movements. TD movements sometimes resolve simply by reducing the dose of medication, and there are now several prescription medications available to treat TD. We used to worry a lot about TD because some people who developed it seemed to continue to have these movements even after they stopped taking the medication. More recent research shows that most TD symptoms *do* eventually go away with time. Also, atypical antipsychotic medications only rarely cause TD.

I want to emphasize that extrapyramidal symptoms are usually easily treated and are not dangerous. But the symptoms of bipolar disorder that antipsychotic medications treat *are* extremely dangerous. These medications are powerful agents, and they need to be used carefully and for the shortest period possible. For the present, at least, they are nearly irreplaceable in treating the most dangerous and most terrible symptoms of severe mania and psychotic depression.

ANTIDEPRESSANT MEDICATIONS

Psychiatrists have debated the role of antidepressant medications in treating the depression of bipolar disorder for decades. This is because these medications can push a person with bipolar disorder from depression into a manic state. Also, in some people, antidepressants seem to increase the cycling of their illness.

However, despite the risks associated with antidepressants for people with bipolar illness, some people appear to benefit from them and can take them safely. Unfortunately, we don't yet have any way of identifying those individuals, so caution is the motto when it comes to prescribing these drugs.

The antidepressants can be divided into groups according to what chemical effects they have on the brain, making for some tongue-twisting labels. By and large, their effects are on *neurotransmitters*, the chemical messengers that that brain cells (*neurons*) use to communicate with each other.

Selective Serotonin Reuptake Inhibitors (SSRIs)

As their name indicates, these medications work through serotonin circuits in the brain. The first SSRI, fluoxetine (Prozac), was introduced in 1988. The SSRIs were a tremendous improvement on older antidepressants (table 4.2). Unlike those drugs, they have fewer side effects, are essentially non-toxic, and are easier to dose. A Prozac capsule showed up on the covers of *Newsweek* and *New York* magazines, and the drug was featured in countless other magazine and newspaper articles.

The side-effect profile of SSRIs is very benign. Because of this, they are usually considered first-line treatment. Thus, if a prescriber decides that a patient may benefit from taking an antidepressant, they will often prescribe an SSRI.

Nausea and headaches are the most common side effects. These usually go away after a few days. If they do not, restarting the medication at a lower dose and increasing it slowly often solves the problem. SSRIs have a caffeine-like effect in some people.

Table 4.2. Selective serotonin reuptake inhibitors (SSRIs)

Pharmaceutical name	Brand name(s)
Citalopram	Celexa (Cipramil)
Escitalopram	Lexapro (Cipralex)
Fluoxetine	Prozac, Sarafem (Erocap, Fluohexal, Lovan, Zactin, and others)
Fluvoxamine	Luvox
Paroxetine	Paxil, Paxil CR* (Aropax, Seroxat, and others)
Sertraline	Zoloft (Altruline, Aremis, Gladem, Besitran, Lustral, Sealdin, and others)

Note: Names in parentheses are brands marketed outside the United States.
* Slow-release preparation.

While this energy boost is just what is needed by some people with depression, others feel unpleasantly nervous or "wired." Many individuals report that SSRIs seem to curb their appetite and notice some weight loss after they begin taking an SSRI. Weight gain can also be a problem, however.

If side effects are going to occur, people usually notice them immediately. SSRI side effects don't sneak up on a person who has been on an SSRI for weeks or months.

About one-third of people taking an SSRI notice a change in sexual functioning—specifically, a noticeable decrease in sexual interest (loss of libido) or difficulty reaching or inability to reach orgasm. Various strategies are available for dealing with these problems when they occur, so they should be reported to the physician. Weekend "vacations" from medication can help. The addition of other drugs that seem to block these effects can also eliminate sexual side effects. Still, sometimes a switch to an antidepressant in another class is the only solution.

Selective Serotonin-Norepinephrine Reuptake Inhibitors (SNRIs)

As you might guess from the name of this group of antidepressants, their activity in the brain involves effects on two systems: serotonin circuits and norepinephrine circuits (table 4.3).

The side-effect profile of the SNRIs is similar to that of the SSRIs. There are indications that the *discontinuation syndrome* for SNRIs can be more severe than for SSRIs.

Table 4.3. Selective serotonin-norepinephrine reuptake inhibitors (SNRIs)

Pharmaceutical name	Brand name(s)
Desvenlafaxine	Pristiq
Duloxetine	Cymbalta (Irenka, Xeristar, Yentreve, and others)
Levomilnacipran	Fetzima
Milnacipran†	Savella†
Venlafaxine	Effexor, Effexor XR* (Efexor, Efexor-XR,* and others)

Note: Names in parentheses are brands marketed outside the United States.

* Slow-release preparation.

† FDA-labeled only for treatment of fibromyalgia.

Tricyclic Antidepressants

Some of the first antidepressant medications to be developed are in this class. These drugs are called *tricyclics* because of the three rings in their chemical structure. The common tricyclics are listed in table 4.4.

The principal reason that tricyclic antidepressants are now less frequently prescribed is because they have many noticeable side effects. As with all medications, some people can take tricyclics easily and without unpleasant side effects. But many people have to put up with a few days or even weeks of troublesome side effects to get the benefits. Fortunately, all the side effects are dose-related, and most are temporary.

Antidepressant Discontinuation Syndrome

You should never stop taking an antidepressant suddenly, especially if you have been taking a higher dose. Doing so runs the risk of developing a collection of uncomfortable symptoms that have been called *discontinuation syndrome*. Fortunately, preventing the problem is straightforward and simply done by tapering the medication slowly. The antidote to the syndrome is also simple: restart the medicine, and then taper more slowly.

Some medications cause more symptoms than others. The SNRIs can be especially troublesome in this regard, while some newer agents, like vortioxetine, rarely cause any discontinuation symptoms.

Symptoms of antidepressant discontinuation syndrome include the following:

- Flu-like symptoms (lethargy, fatigue, headache, achiness, sweating)

- Insomnia (with vivid dreams or nightmares)

- Nausea (sometimes vomiting)

- Imbalance (dizziness, vertigo, light-headedness)

- Sensory disturbances ("brain zaps," "tingling," "electric-like" or "shock-like" sensations)

- Feeling overstimulated (anxiety, irritability, agitation, jerkiness)

Tricyclics block another of the body's chemical messengers in the part of the nervous system that regulates many "automatic" functions of the body, such as digestion. These side effects include a slowing down of the gastrointestinal tract, causing constipation and dry mouth. This system also controls the focusing of the lens of the eye and emptying of the urinary bladder, and tricyclics can cause blurry vision and urination difficulties. Tricyclics also cause weight gain in many people.

Tricyclics are toxic and overdoses can be deadly. Although the lethal overdose is up to twenty times the standard dose for an adult, children are more sensitive to the harmful effects of these drugs. Just a handful of tablets can be fatal in a small child. For this reason, tricyclic medications must be carefully safeguarded in households with children.

Table 4.4. Tricyclic antidepressants

Pharmaceutical name	Brand name
Amitriptyline	Elavil
Amoxapine	Asendin
Clomipramine	Anafranil
Desipramine	Norpramin
Doxepin	Sinequan
Imipramine	Tofranil
Maprotiline	Ludiomil
Nortriptyline	Pamelor
Protriptyline	Vivactil

More Antidepressants

Since the early 1990s, many other new antidepressants have come onto the market that do not fall into any of the preceding categories. Since most of these pharmaceuticals don't share many features, there is no good class name. However, you'll sometimes see many of them listed as *atypical* or *second-generation antidepres-*

sants (table 4.5). The side-effect profiles of these medications vary widely. Some have a profile like that of tricyclics, and others like that of SSRIs.

Table 4.5. Second-generation antidepressants

Pharmaceutical name	Brand name(s)
Agomelatine*	(Melitor, Thymanax, Valdoxan)
Bupropion	Wellbutrin, Wellbutrin SR, Wellbutrin XL
Mirtazapine	Remeron
Vilazodone	Viibryd
Vortioxetine	Trintellix

Note: Names in parentheses are brands marketed outside the United States.
* Not available in the United States.

Monoamine Oxidase Inhibitors (MAOIs)

In the early 1950s, a new drug for tuberculosis was observed to cause mood elevation in some people who took it for their lung disease. Years later, numerous research papers confirmed the therapeutic effects of this medication, iproniazid, in people suffering from depression. Shortly afterward, researchers discovered that iproniazid blocks (or *inhibits*) an enzyme in the body called *monoamine oxidase* (MAO). The name for this class of pharmaceuticals comes from this effect and they are called *monoamine oxidase inhibitors*, or *MAOIs* (table 4.6).

In addition to their effects on the brain, some MAOIs also affect a form of the MAO enzyme present in the gut. Tyramine, a chemical present in some foods, has adrenaline-like effects on blood pressure and heart rate. MAO usually deactivates tyramine in the gut before it gets to the bloodstream. However, in people taking MAOI antidepressants, the MAO in their gut has been blocked by the medication, and the tyramine gets through. Tyramine is present in high enough concentrations in some foods for its adrenaline-like effects to cause dangerous cardiovascular problems in

Table 4.6. Monoamine oxidase inhibitors (MAOIs)

Pharmaceutical name	Brand name(s)
Phenelzine	Nardil
Selegiline	Eldepryl, Emsam transdermal system*
Tranylcypromine	Parnate

* The selegiline patch.

individuals taking MAOIs. Some pharmaceuticals, including the ingredients of many over-the-counter remedies, also have adrenaline-like effects. Therefore, people taking certain MAOIs need to observe specific dietary restrictions. Even more importantly, they must *carefully* read the labels of any over-the-counter medication they are considering. Better yet, consult the pharmacist before taking any pharmaceutical you buy over the counter if you take an MAOI.

One MAOI does not affect the MAO in the gut, and tyramine and other problematic substances don't get past it. This drug is *selegiline* and is available as a patch. The selegiline patch is a way to take an MAOI with fewer side effects and less worry about tyramine-rich foods.

MAOIs can be stimulating and cause insomnia. Dizzy spells, especially when one suddenly gets up from lying down, can occur. Weight gain and sexual dysfunction are other side effects.

Because of these issues, MAOIs are most often prescribed to people who have failed to benefit from other antidepressants. This said, they are sometimes uniquely effective. Indeed, they are "miracle drugs" for some people.

TREATING BIPOLAR DEPRESSION

Taking antidepressants is risky for people with bipolar disorder. There is good evidence that they do not help most people in the long term and may even make things worse.

The observation that antidepressants can cause manic symptoms in people with bipolar disorder has been confirmed again and again. Perhaps more worrisome is the observation that antidepressants may cause an acceleration of the illness in some individuals. Some people with bipolar disorder experience increased cycling of their mood episodes and even switch to rapid cycling.

In the late 1990s, the National Institute of Mental Health sponsored a large, multicenter study of the treatment of bipolar disorder called the Systematic Treatment Enhancement Program for Bipolar Disorder (STEP-BD). This study enrolled more than four thousand people with bipolar disorder and followed them over several years while they received treatment. One surprising finding was in a subgroup of 350 patients who developed depression during the study. About half of these patients were then prescribed an antidepressant in addition to their mood stabilizer. At the same time, the others stayed on the mood stabilizer alone. At the end of about six months, antidepressant medications appeared to have offered no benefit whatsoever. Another surprise was that the patients who took an antidepressant had no more problems with manic symptoms than those who took only a mood stabilizer. Now, this seems to fly in the face of decades of research and clinical experience. It demonstrates what I said at the beginning of this chapter—that some people with bipolar disorder need, benefit from, and can safely take antidepressants. The problem is that we have no way of identifying the people in this sub-group. However, it makes the point strongly that these individuals are the exception, not the rule. Most people with bipolar disorder should probably avoid taking antidepressant medications.

Antidepressants and the Risk of Mania

One of the first research papers on an antidepressant, "The Treatment of Depressive States with G22355, Imipramine Hydrochloride," reported a potential problem. The author noted that "in individuals who are predisposed," the drug could "give rise to manic-like states or even a manic state." This observation has been thoroughly confirmed since this paper appeared in 1958. The "predisposed individuals" are now recognized to be people with bipolar disorder.

It is also clear that antidepressants do not have this effect on all people with bipolar disorder. A rule of thumb seems to be that the more severe the manic or hypomanic symptoms an individual has had previously, the higher the risk of developing manic symptoms from taking an antidepressant. Thus, people with bipolar I are at higher risk than are people with bipolar II.

Some antidepressants are more likely than others to trigger manic symptoms in a person with bipolar disorder. This is one proposed ranking of this risk:

Higher risk   Tricyclic antidepressants
of mania   SNRIs
   SSRIs
Lower risk   Bupropion

R. M. Post, L. L. Altshuler, M. A. Frye, T. Suppes, A. J. Rush, P. E. Keck Jr., S. L. McElroy, et al., "Rate of Switch in Bipolar Patients Prospectively Treated with Second-Generation Antidepressants as Augmentation to Mood Stabilizers," *Bipolar Disorders* 3, no. 5 (2001): 259–65.

Studies on mania and rapid cycling triggered by antidepressants indicate that some people are at more risk than others for these problems. Unfortunately, it is not possible to say with certainty who is and who is not at risk. People with bipolar I seem to be at greater risk than those with bipolar II, and women seem to be at greater risk than men. People who already have a history of more rapid cycling also appear to be at greater risk. Moreover, a few studies indicate that some antidepressant medications seem to be safer than others. Some drugs are less likely to precipitate mania (and, by implication, are perhaps less likely to increase cycling).

Perhaps more than any other treatment issue, the questions surrounding the use of antidepressants in bipolar disorder emphasize the need to individualize treatment for every person. There are no hard-and-fast rules for when, why, or how to use an antidepressant for people with bipolar disorder. Patients and physicians need to communicate clearly and honestly about every aspect of symptoms and treatment to achieve the best treatment outcome.

Key Takeaways about Antidepressants

❖ *The prescription of antidepressants to people with bipolar disorder is controversial and not without risk.*

❖ *There is significant research evidence that antidepressants can trigger mania, induce mixed states, and increase mood cycling in some people with bipolar disorder.*

❖ *One of the results of the STEP-BD study was that as a group, people with bipolar disorder do not benefit from antidepressants in the long term. However, there is likely a subgroup of bipolar individuals who benefit from and can safely take antidepressants.*

Beware of ACID

Another instructive finding from the STEP-BD study was that some people with bipolar disorder who took antidepressants and appeared to recover from depression developed several problems. They started having more insomnia problems, feelings of tense uneasiness that psychiatrists call "dysphoria," along with smoldering irritability. The STEP-BD researchers referred to this set of symptoms as "ACID," short for *antidepressant-associated chronic irritable dysphoria*. They found that these people were often quite impaired by these symptoms. The researchers already suspected that antidepressants were the cause of this problem, so they looked through the records of STEP-BD patients with this trio: chronic irritability, dysphoria, and sleep disturbances. They also noted who had or had not taken an antidepressant along with their mood stabilizer. The results were unequivocal. They found that the individuals with ACID who had taken an antidepressant outnumbered those taking only a mood stabilizer by ten to one.

Post et al., "Rate of Switch"; and R. S. El-Mallakh, S. N. Ghaemi, K. Sagduyu, M. E. Thase, S. R. Wisniewski, A. A. Nierenberg, H. W. Zhang, T. A. Pardo, and G. Sachs (STEP-BD Investigators), "Antidepressant-Associated Chronic Irritable Dysphoria (ACID) in STEP-BD Patients," *Journal of Affective Disorders* 111, nos. 2–3 (2008): 372–7. https://doi.org/10.1016/j.jad.2008.03.025.

CHAPTER 5

More Medications, Hormones, and Nutritional Supplements

Many other pharmaceuticals have proven to be helpful in the treatment of bipolar disorder. Some are *symptomatic treatments*, meaning that they treat symptoms rather than the underlying condition and are usually used for only a short time. Others are medications that affect functioning in another body system that is important for normal mood regulation.

Sleeplessness and anxiety are common problems for people with mood disorders. Sleep deprivation is often acutely destabilizing for people with mood disorders. Anxiety raises the levels of stress hormones in the body, which can also be destabilizing. Therefore, keeping these uncomfortable symptoms in check is an essential part of staying well.

MEDICATIONS FOR ANXIETY AND SLEEP DISTURBANCES

Benzodiazepine Medications

The development of benzodiazepine medications in the 1970s represented a significant advance in treating psychiatric symptoms. They are highly effective for treating anxiety and insomnia and, in higher doses, are safe and effective sedatives. If this sounds too good to be true and you're wondering if there's a hidden drawback, there is. Some people can misuse benzodiazepines. It's possible to become psychologically dependent and even physically addicted to them. (Withdrawal symptoms in people taking high doses of these medications can include serious problems such as seizures.) Also, their effectiveness against insomnia often wanes after several weeks of use. For these reasons, benzodiazepines are best thought of as temporary measures. Nevertheless, some people benefit from and can safely take them over the longer term (table 5.1).

Benzodiazepines have two primary uses in treating bipolar disorder: they are used to treat people who are very sick and treat people who are doing very well.

In people with acute mania, the short-acting benzodiazepine lorazepam (Ativan) can be an effective short-term tranquilizer, especially in combination with a typical antipsychotic medication like haloperidol (Haldol). This combination is familiar to psychiatrists working in emergency settings because it works quickly and effectively calms even the most agitated individuals. A person with acute mania, perhaps delusional and agitated, who hasn't slept for days can be asleep less than an hour after receiving this combination, especially by injection. The longer-acting benzodiazepine clonazepam (Klonopin) has also been used for this purpose and extensively studied for treating manic symptoms.

Table 5.1. Benzodiazepine medications

Pharmaceutical name	Brand name
Alprazolam	Xanax
Chlordiazepoxide	Librium
Clonazepam	Klonopin
Clorazepate	Tranxene
Diazepam	Valium
Lorazepam	Ativan

Note: These medications are best thought of as temporary agents and are frequently prescribed for occasional "as-needed" use.

These medications are not mood stabilizers and are not effective in treating hallucinations or delusions, but as anti-anxiety medications, they are unsurpassed. Before effective psychiatric drugs became available, people with severe mania died of the physical stress caused by the manic state. By simply slowing people with mania down for a few hours or days until antipsychotic medications and mood-stabilizing medications start working, benzodiazepines can be lifesaving.

At the other end of the spectrum of illness severity, people who are not having severe mood symptoms can safely take these medications in the short term for anxiety symptoms and insomnia. During periods of unavoidable psychological stress, such as after the death of a loved one, benzodiazepine medications can help with insomnia. They can also lessen the psychological tension that may bring on mood symptoms in people with bipolar disorder. It's important to emphasize that these medications should *not* be substitutes for making changes to chronically stressful situations. A person who finds that they feel the need to take a sedative to deal with everyday problems is well on their way to psychological dependence on tranquilizers, medication abuse, and addiction.

Benzodiazepines are also used to treat anxiety disorders. The connections between mood disorders and anxiety disorders are poorly understood. There are certainly some people who need treatment for both. The treatment of panic disorder and other severe anxiety disorders sometimes involves taking benzodiazepine medications on a longer-term basis. Still, prolonged use of benzodiazepines is the exception rather than the rule in treating bipolar disorders.

Most people can take these medications safely, but a minority get into serious trouble with them. When taken on a long-term basis, they can produce *tolerance*: needing higher doses to get the same effect. However, escalating doses can quickly lead to psychological and physical addiction.

The elderly are especially prone to problems with these medications, which increase the risk of memory problems, falls, hip fractures, and motor vehicle accidents.

Benzodiazepine medications are usually safe and effective, especially in the short term. Still, there are significant risks, especially when taken for prolonged periods or in high doses.

Other Medications for Anxiety

Two medications developed as a treatment for epilepsy have proved to be helpful for people with anxiety problems. Both are active in a neuroreceptor system known to be involved with anxiety, the GABA pathway (for gamma-aminobutyric acid). Their names reflect this: *gabapentin* (Neurontin) and pre*gabalin* (Lyrica). These medications have several advantages for treating the anxiety that can be associated with bipolar disorder. The first is that there is little or no risk of developing a psychological dependence on them. Gabapentin is not a "controlled substance" in FDA parlance. Although pregabalin is a controlled substance, it has the lowest possible risk rating: schedule V. (Other schedule V drugs include cough medicines with small amounts of codeine). Also, gabapentin and pregabalin do not lose their effectiveness when taken long-term. For these reasons, they can be helpful for people with prolonged anxiety problems that have no clear cause. This pattern is often called "generalized anxiety."

"Z-drugs"

This group of medications gets its name from the fact that several of them start with the letter Z. Zolpidem was the first of these medications, introduced in 1992, and zaleplon followed soon after. Zopiclone is another, though it is not available in the United States. The Z-drugs were derived from benzodiazepines and share many of their features. However, they are more specific to sleep circuitry than are benzodiazepines. These medications are prescribed almost exclusively for insomnia because they are absorbed rapidly and the body gets rid of them quickly. These features make them nearly ideal sleep medications. They work fast and don't

Table 5.2. "Z-drugs"

Pharmaceutical name	Brand name
Eszopiclone	Lunesta
Zaleplon	Sonata
Zopiclone*	Imovane
Zolpidem	Ambien, Ambien CR, Intermezzo, and others

* Not commercially available in the United States.

stay around too long, meaning that a next-morning "hangover" feeling is uncommon. The Z-drugs are somewhat less likely than benzodiazepines to cause rebound insomnia when people stop taking them and therefore are less likely to cause dependence. They are also less likely to lose their effectiveness over time (tolerance) (table 5.2).

Like benzodiazepines, however, they can be misused. People can become addicted to them, though this is rare unless they are taken in much higher doses than recommended.

The elderly are more sensitive to these medications. As with benzodiazepines, they increase the risk of falls, hip fractures, and motor vehicle accidents.

Melatonin

Melatonin can be thought of as a sleep hormone. Most of the body's melatonin is produced in and released into the bloodstream from the pineal gland, a small organ located deep within the brain. It also happens to be synthesized by various plants and is found in the seeds of sunflowers and coriander.

Although melatonin can help treat sleep problems, it is not a sedative or "sleeping pill." It doesn't put you to sleep by tamping down brain functioning like benzodiazepines and Z-drugs. Instead, melatonin tells the brain's sleep center that it's time to start the sleep process. Thus, melatonin should be considered a sleep *regulator*.

Taking melatonin essentially boosts the brain's "go to sleep" signal—and in a very natural way, as it is the same molecule that the body produces. Taking melatonin has been shown to improve the onset, duration, and quality of sleep. I often recommend melatonin as the first thing to try for sleep problems, as it has none of the problems associated with benzodiazepines or Z-drugs. Melatonin does not cause tolerance, dependence, or adverse effects on alertness or mood the following day (the hangover effect). Most sleep experts suggest taking 1–3 milligrams (mg) of immediate-release melatonin (and avoiding slow-release preparations) two hours before bedtime for insomnia. This dose and timing appear to do the best job of mimicking the normal physiological cycle of the body.

There is a pharmaceutical that mimics the effects of melatonin called *ramelteon* (Rozerem). Ramelteon has been shown to be "modestly effective" in improving sleep factors, but whether it is superior to melatonin has not been tested.

THYROID HORMONES

The thyroid gland plays a vital role in the body's energy regulation. Too little thyroid gland activity leads to sluggishness and weight gain. Too much leads to metabolic overdrive—rapid pulse, nervous energy, and anxiety. While the precise role of thyroid hormones in mood regulation remains unclear, it's clear that normal thyroid functioning is essential for the effective treatment of mood disorders. Put another way, if a person's mood symptoms don't respond to the usual treatments or if a treatment that has been effective seems to lose its effectiveness, a thyroid problem, especially abnormally low thyroid functioning (hypothyroidism), should be suspected.

Several studies have shown that hypothyroidism is surprisingly common in people with rapid-cycling bipolar disorder. One group of scientists looked for thyroid abnormalities in stored blood samples from almost four thousand patients hospitalized for psychiatric problems. They found a high association between thyroid abnormalities and a diagnosis of rapid-cycling bipolar disorder.

But it is also clear that some people with bipolar disorder whose thyroid hormone levels are in the "normal range" can benefit from treatment with thyroid medications. Studies have demonstrated that many people with bipolar depression symptoms that are not responding to treatment have thyroid function that is "normal" by the usual criteria. However, a closer look reveals that their thyroid hormone levels are in what might be called the "low normal" or even "barely normal" range. It may be that individuals with depression need a higher level of thyroid hormones than those who are not depressed. Perhaps the extra thyroid hormone somehow makes these people more responsive to other treatments. People who have a partial response to lithium or other mood stabilizers may have better control of their mood symptoms if they take a small dose of thyroid replacement hormone, even if their thyroid hormone levels are "normal." As a paper on treating rapid-cycling bipolar disorder put it, "Normal thyroid [blood test results] should not discourage the clinician from pursuing thyroid supplementation" in people with bipolar disorder.

Notice that I haven't used the term *thyroid medication* in this discussion. That is because it has been possible for many years to synthetically produce the same molecules that the thyroid gland itself naturally produces. (Hence the brand name, Synthroid, of the most commonly prescribed brand of levothyroxine.) What dose of hormone to prescribe is determined by measuring hormone levels in the blood, which should be done at least several times a year for anyone who takes a thyroid hormone replacement.

HERBAL PREPARATIONS AND NUTRITIONAL SUPPLEMENTS

There are some nutrients that we must include in our diet to remain healthy. These are compounds that our body cannot manufacture but are nevertheless necessary for normal cellular functioning. The most familiar of these are, of course, the *vitamins*. Unless we eat foods that contain the vitamins we need, we become seriously ill. Scurvy, beriberi, and pellagra are three illnesses—now, thankfully, unfamiliar—caused by deficiencies of vitamin C, vitamin B1, and niacin, respectively.

There are other naturally occurring substances that our bodies are not very good at producing that are important for health. *Essential fatty acids* are excellent examples of these substances. These are fat molecules found in some vegetables and other plant sources (such as flaxseed) and in large amounts in some fish. Nutritionists have long touted the health benefits of diets rich in seafood. The lower incidence of breast cancer and heart disease in the Japanese population has been attributed to such a diet.

There are other substances derived from plants that can be beneficial for bodily functioning. As a group, these are often referred to as "herbal supplements," "botanicals," or "nutraceuticals."

The FDA tends to be reluctant to regulate naturally occurring substances as pharmaceuticals. Instead, the FDA considers them "nutritional supplements." They are regulated as foods, even if the manufacturing process occurs in a pharmaceutical manufacturing facility and doesn't involve food or plants or anything one would think of as "natural."

Omega-3 Fatty Acids and Fish Oil

Some evidence suggests that essential fatty acids, especially a subgroup called *omega-3 fatty acids*, may be helpful in the treatment of bipolar disorder. A review article that analyzed five studies in people with bipolar depression concluded that there is "strong evidence that bipolar depression may be improved by the adjunctive use of omega-3." Studies of omega-3 in mania have not shown any benefit.

Omega-3 fatty acid therapy is an adjunctive treatment (a treatment given alongside primary treatment) for bipolar disorder when added to other agents such as lithium. It is *not* a substitute for proven treatments. However, given the apparent low risk of these compounds, some people will want to explore the supplementation of standard therapies for mood disorders with omega-3 preparations under the supervision of one's physician.

N-Acetyl Cysteine

Although oxygen is a vital ingredient for biological functioning, it is highly reactive chemically. It can combine with just about anything in a reaction called oxygenation, often with untoward results. When oxygen rapidly combines with the organic compounds in gasoline, we call it "fire." When oxygen combines with various molecules in the body, a much less dramatic but still harmful process occurs called *oxidative stress*. Plants and animals all make substances in their tissues that prowl about, scooping up these damaging oxygen-containing molecules when they occur. You can think of oxidative stress as a kind of biological overheating, requiring *anti*oxidants to step in and cool things down. NAC is an integral part of our antioxidant system. Several studies have demonstrated that it can be a helpful add-on medication for people with bipolar disorder.

Like omega-3, NAC is an adjunctive medication, the benefits of which should be considered promising rather than firmly established. Nevertheless, it is an option some may wish to explore— again, with the guidance of their physician.

St. John's Wort

Hypericum perforatum, commonly known as St. John's wort, is one of about three hundred species of shrubby perennial plants of the genus *Hypericum*. Herbalists have recommended teas and other St. John's wort extracts for centuries to treat everything from insomnia to the painful viral skin infection called shingles.

In the late 1990s, there was a great deal of interest in St. John's wort as a treatment for depression. Careful study since then has not borne out the initial claims of benefit, especially for people with severe depression. However, it is enough of an antidepressant to trigger manic symptoms in some individuals. I think it's fair to say that St. John's wort isn't good enough as an antidepressant to help people with bipolar disorder, but it's enough of an antidepressant to cause problems for them. So it is best avoided, except perhaps in the garden.

Key Takeaways

❖ *Benzodiazepines and Z-drugs are often prescribed to individuals with bipolar disorder to treat insomnia and anxiety. Although effective, there are risks associated with them, especially if used in the long term.*

❖ *Melatonin is the body's sleep hormone, and taking it as a supplement can be effective for insomnia.*

❖ *Robust thyroid functioning is necessary for mood disorder treatments to be effective; this sometimes means taking thyroid hormones.*

❖ *Several nutraceuticals and botanicals have been shown to help people with bipolar disorder as add-ons to medications. St. John's wort, however, should be avoided, as it has been reported to trigger manic symptoms.*

CHAPTER 6

Brain Stimulation Treatments

Several medical treatments for mood disorders use tiny electrical impulses to stimulate brain areas involved in mood control. One of them has been around for many decades. Several others are quite new. Yet others are still investigational treatments. All take advantage of the fact that electrical impulses increase or decrease the activity level of brain cells.

In the oldest of these techniques, electroconvulsive therapy, an electrical current is applied directly to the scalp while the patient is under general anesthesia. Newer methods use much smaller electrical impulses and require no anesthesia. Although the details of how these treatments work are still far from certain, they all appear to treat mood disorders by affecting the levels of electrical activity in some regions of the brain—specifically, the brain areas that are underactive or overactive during episodes of abnormal mood. They bring activity levels into a more normal balance, in much the same way that tiny electrical impulses regulate heart rhythms in individuals who have a cardiac pacemaker.

ELECTROCONVULSIVE THERAPY

ECT is only rarely used to treat people with bipolar disorder. But for those few people for whom nothing else is effective, it can be nothing short of lifesaving. It is a valuable therapeu-

tic tool for any person with bipolar disorder who is extremely sick and seems to be getting sicker despite aggressive treatment with medication. It is perhaps the most effective treatment for severe depression and severe mania. It often works more quickly than medications.

The development of modern ECT, like so many other treatments in psychiatry, was discovered almost accidentally. In the early 1930s, the Hungarian physician Ladislas J. von Meduna proposed that people who suffered from epilepsy were somehow protected from developing schizophrenia. Modern research has shown that this is not the case. Still, von Meduna conducted animal experiments, attempting to find a way to artificially produce seizure activity. He thought that this might be a way to treat the symptoms of schizophrenia. In 1935, he published a paper reporting a dramatic improvement in psychiatric symptoms after artificially inducing seizures in several patients. He thought that these patients had schizophrenia, although, in retrospect, at least some probably had severe mood disorders with psychotic symptoms. Several years later, two Italian psychiatrists reported that they had produced seizures in dogs by briefly passing a low-voltage electrical current through the skull using electrodes applied to the scalp. Ugo Cerletti and Lucio Bini later administered these treatments to several patients with "schizophrenia" and also reported remarkable success.

Although people with schizophrenia do often show improvement in some of their symptoms after these treatments (catatonia is one such symptom), it quickly became apparent that it was the people with severe depression who showed the most dramatic improvement—an improvement that was little short of miraculous.

The Ups and Downs of ECT:
Why the Bad Rap?

In his famous textbook of psychiatry, Emil Kraepelin described people in a catatonic state from psychotic depression: "The patients lie in bed taking no interest in anything. They betray no pronounced emotion; they are mute, inaccessible; they pass their [bowel movements] under them; they stare straight in front of them with [a] vacant expression . . . like a mask and with wide-open eyes."* In the 1940s, psychiatrists observed that giving these people "electroshock" treatments entirely relieved their terrible symptoms within a matter of days. At the time, the most recent significant breakthrough in the treatment of psychiatric problems had been in 1906, when the Wassermann test for syphilis was developed. That development now seemed almost insignificant compared with this astonishing, even miraculous new therapeutic technique. Naturally, interest in ECT spread quickly around the globe.

But ECT's success was also nearly its downfall. Like many other seemingly miraculous treatments, psychiatrists overprescribed it at first. It probably was administered to many hundreds of people it had little chance of helping.

It's important to remember, however, that those were desperate times in psychiatry. With the discovery of antipsychotic medications nearly a decade away, and the discovery of antidepressants almost two decades into the future, a "little chance" of helping was better than no chance at all.

In the first decade or so after its development, ECT could have some very serious complications. An epileptic seizure can be a violent event: all the muscles of the body contract simultaneously for a few moments, sometimes with such force that broken bones result. Breathing stops as well, and heart-rhythm irregularities can occur. The nearly indiscriminate overprescribing of a therapy with potentially severe side effects unsurprisingly led to a backlash. Although modern anesthetic techniques had made ECT safer, and more careful research determined which psychiatric disorders the treatment helped with, the damage to ECT's reputation was already done. (The famous depiction of ECT in the film *One Flew over the Cuckoo's Nest*, awarded the Oscar for Best Picture in 1975, which portrayed ECT as it would have been administered circa 1945, certainly didn't help.) State hospitals drew up regulations sharply curtailing its use, and legislation was briefly in effect in California banning the procedure altogether.

Fortunately, the pendulum has swung back to the center. ECT is now safer than most surgical procedures, side effects are minimal, and guidelines for prescribing it for a patient have been clarified. A 1980 survey of 166 ECT patients reported that about half thought a trip to the dentist was more unpleasant than an electroconvulsive treatment.[†]

---

*Kraepelin, *Manic-Depressive Insanity*, 97.

[†] C. P. L. Freeman and R. E. Kendell, "ECT I: Patients' Experiences and Attitudes," *British Journal of Psychiatry* 137, no. 1 (1980): 8–16. https://doi.org/10.1192/bjp.137.1.8.

Modern ECT

Since its introduction in the 1940s, there have been vast improvements in ECT techniques that have dramatically reduced side effects and adverse events. There have been changes to minimize the electrical energy delivered. Perhaps even more importantly, modern anesthesia essentially eliminates physical side-effect problems.

About the only people who absolutely must not receive ECT are the few individuals with such severe medical conditions that they cannot tolerate even ten to fifteen minutes of general anesthesia—for example, people with severe cardiac or lung diseases. ECT is safe to administer to elderly people and during pregnancy.

The Experience of ECT

Most psychiatric hospitals have specialized treatment suites for ECT; in general hospitals, it is often administered in the recovery room of the hospital's surgical suite (the area where patients wake up from surgery).

The crucial anesthetic advance for ECT was the introduction in the 1950s of agents called *muscle relaxants*, or, more appropriately, *neuromuscular blocking agents*. These drugs temporarily paralyze the patient by blocking nerve-fiber signals to the muscles, preventing the violent muscle contractions during seizures that characterized early ECT use.

After an intravenous medication is given to put the patient to sleep, the neuromuscular blocking agent is given through the IV. This temporarily paralyzes the patient's muscles. Electrode disks similar to those used for cardiac defibrillation are applied to the scalp. Modern ECT equipment designed for the purpose delivers a precisely timed and measured electrical stimulus. In *bilateral* treatments, the treating physician applies an electrode over each temple. In *unilateral* treatments, wherein the object is to stimulate only half of the brain, one electrode is placed in the middle of the forehead or the crown of the head and the other at the temple. (Unilateral treatment causes less post-ECT confusion and memory problems. They are now prescribed almost exclusively, although people for whom unilateral treatments are ineffective often switch to bilateral treatments.)

The electrical stimulus is applied for two to eight seconds, triggering seizure activity in the brain. Because of the muscle relaxant, the "seizure" in modern ECT is pretty much an electrical event only, with few or no jerking movements such as those that usually characterize seizures. For this reason, it is called a *modified seizure*. The entire treatment lasts about twenty to thirty minutes. Most of this time is the ten minutes or so it takes to administer general anesthesia before the actual treatment and another ten minutes for the patient to awaken from it.

The ECT equipment also records an electroencephalogram (a measurement of the brain's electrical activity), allowing the physician to monitor the seizure activity, which usually lasts less than a minute. There might be some muscle contractions observed during this time, but the muscle relaxant keeps the patient nearly motionless. There is usually a quickening of the heart rate and an increase in blood pressure. These changes also signal that the "seizure" has occurred. The anesthetist uses a face-mask breathing device to deliver oxygen until the patient wakes up five or ten minutes later, and the treatment is over.

ECT Side Effects

The most troublesome side effect of ECT relates to its impact on memory. In a recent study, about a quarter (twenty-six percent) of people receiving ECT reported memory problems immediately after a course of ECT. Fortunately, most studies show that this is a temporary problem that resolves in several weeks for most people.

There are two types of memory problems that ECT can cause. The first is a problem with the kind of memory needed to get places and find things (called *visuospatial memory*). The other is a problem with the memory of things that have happened (called *autobiographical memory*). In a famous article in the *British Journal of Psychiatry*, a practicing psychiatrist who received ECT for depression described his experience with the first type of memory problem. For several weeks after his course of ECT, he could no longer remember how to get where he needed to go using the London subway system. He suddenly found that he had forgotten where the different lines went and needed to consult station maps, even for routine trips that he had taken for years. After a time, everything became familiar again. He was knowledgeable enough about what was going on to find the whole thing amusing rather than a source of worry (or at least, that's what he wrote in the article). But what happens if people are not prepared to expect this possible side effect? In that case, they can be quite alarmed when they return home and find their house oddly unfamiliar. Maybe they can't lay their hands on their favorite frying pan or remember where in the world those darn hedge trimmers are. Getting lost going to the supermarket? Not at all uncommon—at least for a few weeks. The experience of the English psychiatrist is a reminder that being forewarned and prepared for these potential problems is essential so that if and when they occur, they are not so frightening.

Autobiographical memory, the other type of memory loss that can follow ECT, affects the memory of events occurring during the several weeks when the patient is receiving ECT and sometimes the memories of events before that, a problem called *retrograde amnesia*. People who have completed a course of ECT may say they don't remember checking into the hospital. They might not recollect a home visit or a trip they took with their family during the treatments. This problem seems to be worst just after an individual receives ECT. In a study to better understand these problems, researchers asked forty-three ECT patients about their memory a few weeks after completing a course of ECT. Some patients reported difficulty remembering events for a period of up to two years before their ECT. However, when these patients were tested again seven *months* after their treatment, they had almost completely recovered their distant memories.

ECT for Bipolar Disorder

Electroconvulsive therapy can be thought of as a symptomatic treatment for both phases of bipolar disorder. (A *symptomatic* treatment treats *symptoms* but not the underlying disease).

ECT can quickly interrupt an episode of depression or mania, but its beneficial effect does not always last. This means that medication will still be necessary to sustain the benefit of ECT and to keep the person's mood state stable after finishing the treatments.

ECT is generally considered to be the most effective antidepressant treatment available. Naturally, it should be a treatment consideration whenever a person with bipolar disorder continues to be severely depressed despite aggressive medication treatment. It is also *rapidly* effective. Often, people dramatically improve after just three or four treatments—that is, after five to seven days. People who are seriously contemplating suicide or those who have stopped eating and drinking and are in danger of malnutrition and dehydration—anyone for whom profound depression has become a life-threatening illness—are candidates for ECT. ECT is often used during pregnancy to treat severe bipolar depression because of the risk that many mood-stabilizing medications pose to the fetus. Depression can be highly resistant to antidepressant medications in elderly people. Therefore, experts frequently recommend it as a first-line treatment for severe depression in older people. People with bipolar disorder who are depressed and receive ECT can become slightly hypomanic. When this occurs, it's time to stop the treatments. Unlike antidepressants, ECT does not seem to increase the cycling of the illness. ECT is also a highly effective treatment for mania.

TRANSCRANIAL MAGNETIC STIMULATION (TMS)

Transcranial magnetic stimulation (TMS) is a new brain stimulation technique that effectively treats mood disorders. TMS has a great advantage over ECT in that it is much simpler to administer: the treatment induces no seizure activity, and therefore no anesthesia is necessary. Even more advantageous is that there are almost no side effects.

This novel technique takes advantage of a principle of electromagnetism called *induction* to deliver an electrical stimulus to the brain without applying electrical energy to the scalp (as in ECT). During TMS treatments, the patient sits in a chair that is similar to a dentist's chair. A technician places a TMS device against the patient's head or, with some devices, lowers a "helmet" similar to a hair-dryer hood used in beauty salons over the patient's head. The device delivers pulses of magnetic energy for about twenty to forty minutes. The patient simply sits in the chair, awake and alert throughout the whole procedure. Other than some soreness from muscle stimulation, there appear to be no side effects of any kind.

One of the first studies on TMS in the treatment of depression appeared in the *American Journal of Psychiatry* in 1997. In this study from the National Institute of Mental Health, there was a statistically significant mood improvement in these individuals after TMS treatments but not after the placebo treatments. Several people continued TMS after completing the study and experienced additional clinical improvement in their depressive symptoms. The FDA approved the first TMS device in 2008 and another device in 2013 to treat major depression.

There are many more studies of using TMS in people with unipolar depression than in people with bipolar disorder. Nevertheless, studies of individuals with bipolar disorder have been encouraging.

Over the past ten years or so, TMS has continued to evolve. It has become clear that more magnetic pulses per session are more effective. However, psychiatrists are still learning how best to administer them. The strength of the magnetic stimulation that is most beneficial, the type and exact placement of the coil, the number of magnetic impulses delivered per treatment session, the total number of treatments, and the duration of therapy are all under investigation at various centers around the world.

Further developments in TMS include *theta burst stimulation TMS* (TBS), which combines high-frequency and low-frequency pulses during TMS treatments. TBS treatments last only about five minutes instead of the twenty to forty-five minutes required for regular TMS treatments. Another new variation is *synchronized TMS* (sTMS). Here, the device delivers the magnetic bursts in sync with the patient's brain waves. Both of these investigational treatments use less magnetic energy and appear to be more comfortable for people.

TMS has been a promising development in treating mood disorders and is already opening up a whole new array of treatment options.

TRANSCRANIAL DIRECT CURRENT STIMULATION (tDCS)

This is an investigational treatment in which a small electrical current is delivered using electrodes applied to the scalp's surface. This technique resembles electroconvulsive therapy in that an electrical current is passed directly through the skull, but the current is only a tiny fraction of that used in ECT. Whereas the current delivered by an ECT device is usually 800 milliamperes (mA), tDCS devices deliver only two mA. As with transcranial magnetic stimulation, the patient can remain awake, simply sitting in a chair during the treatments, and no anesthesia is required. These treatments, like TMS, last about twenty minutes and are repeated daily for several weeks. A significant advantage of tDCS over TMS is that the equipment is much simpler and hence less expensive. Several studies of tDCS to treat bipolar disorder have been published, and the results have been encouraging.

Key Takeaways

❖ *Brain stimulation treatments consist of several therapeutic techniques that use electrical energy to stimulate areas of the brain.*

❖ *Electroconvulsive therapy (ECT) has been around the longest, is the most studied, and is considered the most effective. ECT requires general anesthesia and often causes memory problems.*

❖ *Several newer brain stimulation treatments (TMS and tDCS) use much smaller amounts of electrical energy to stimulate the brain. These techniques target the affected areas of the brain more precisely than ECT. Whether these treatments are as effective as ECT remains to be confirmed, but results so far are encouraging.*

CHAPTER 7

Essential Ingredients: Therapy and Counseling

The second leg of the three-legged stool of best practices for treating bipolar disorder is often referred to as "talk therapy"—that is, psychotherapy and counseling. Just as physical therapists play a vital role in helping someone heal from a stroke or a broken limb, psychotherapists play a crucial role in helping someone recover from a mood episode and learn how to live with a long-term illness.

WHAT IS PSYCHOTHERAPY?

Although medical treatments such as pharmaceuticals are the foundation of the treatment of bipolar disorder, counseling and psychotherapy are important, perhaps indispensable, additional therapeutic interventions. The word *psychotherapy* can be translated as "therapy for the mind." (The word *psyche* comes from the Greek word for "mind.") Some people still picture psychotherapy as something that happens in a richly paneled, dimly lit office where a bearded psychiatrist sits taking notes in a high-backed leather chair behind a patient who's lying on a couch and trying to remember what they dreamed about last night. Or perhaps they think of talk-radio therapists, dispensing sound-bite-sized advice to the lovelorn and lonely between car commercials on the AM dial. All of this is psychotherapy of a sort, but the practice of psychotherapy is a well-studied clinical intervention for individuals in psychological distress. It requires years of training and experience to master.

There are many types of counseling and therapy that are enormously helpful in treating bipolar disorder. By reading this book to this point, you've already received several hours of a kind of therapy. You've allowed an objective but sympathetic individual with knowledge and experience about mental illness and psychological processes (that's me) to present facts about bipolar disorder to increase your understanding of the illness. This understanding has, I hope, helped you make sense of your thoughts and feelings about this problem as it affects you. There's even a name for just this sort of treatment—*psychoeducation*—and it has been proven in research studies to reduce illness recurrences, decrease the number and duration of hospitalizations, increase the time to illness relapse, and lead to reduced stigma.

This is, in considerable measure, what psychotherapy is all about: not interpreting dreams, not simply doling out advice, and certainly not supplying all the answers, but providing good, objective information and feedback to help people make sense of their thoughts and feelings. It's been said that psychotherapy benefits people who feel discouraged by helping them to rewrite their life story—for example, to take "I'm just a crazy person" and rewrite that story to "I'm a pretty well-adjusted person who happens to have bipolar disorder."

Brain and Mind

Psychotherapy was developed in the late 1800s by a young neurologist from Vienna whose name is probably familiar to you: Sigmund Freud. Many of Freud's fellow psychiatrists, such as Emil Kraepelin, were caring for seriously ill patients in psychiatric hospitals. Others were working in their laboratories to understand brain disorders like schizophrenia and Alzheimer's disease (named, by the way, after a contemporary of Freud, Dr. Alois Alzheimer). However, the young Dr. Freud saw patients who had symptoms of depression or anxiety but were otherwise living ordinary lives in their community.

Freud spent his lifetime treating and trying to understand people who were unhappy in their relationships, disappointed in themselves for the choices they made, perhaps confused and anxious about decisions they were facing. Freud and his followers developed a large and sophisticated system for understanding human behavior and treatments. This approach consisted of helping people to understand themselves better and to let go of grudges, resentments, and fears rooted in their past. Most importantly, this new kind of psychiatrist helped their patient learn better, more mature strategies to cope with life's challenges. Freud's fundamental insights continue to form the basis for the practice of psychotherapy. Thanks to Freud, we now take for granted that psychological traumas can cause debilitating symptoms like panic attacks, severe depression, and flashbacks. We also take for granted that these symptoms can be effectively treated by talking about the traumatic experiences in a safe, confidential setting with a knowledgeable and supportive professional. This approach to treating psychological problems is directly attributable to Freud.

Freud's approach is now called *dynamic* psychotherapy (or *psychodynamic* psychotherapy) because it understands mental life as a dynamic interplay between emotions and intellect, present circumstances and unconscious memories of past experiences, and many other psychological factors.

The variety of available psychological treatments has broadened tremendously since Freud's time, and they have become much more focused. Sophisticated techniques have been developed that work for particular kinds of problems. Some involve individual sessions with a therapist; others occur in a group setting. Some methods focus on a specific issue, such as marital or family difficulties or addiction. Others concentrate on a particular symptom, such as depression or phobias. Some are designed to last only a few sessions; others are more open-ended. Some are not "therapy" in the traditional sense at all: support groups, made up of individuals who offer guidance and support to each other, don't even include a "therapist." Clinical researchers have, in many cases, determined which psychological treatments work best for which problems.

What Can Therapy Do?

No one today would even think of recommending counseling or therapy as the only treatment for bipolar disorder. But because we have highly effective medications for this illness, some want to turn away from counseling and therapy altogether. Some want to approach the illness as a purely "chemical" problem with a purely "chemical" solution. This is a mistake for several reasons.

First of all, the diagnosis of bipolar disorder is almost always a traumatic event, not only for individuals but also for their family members. In addition to the emotional turmoil that is the symptom of the illness itself, there is an emotional trauma that results from coming face-to-face with one's fears about how this diagnosis will affect their life. Vaguely familiar terms like *manic depression* and all-too-familiar terms like *mental illness* conjure up all sorts of confused and confusing ideas and feelings. "Why has this happened to me?" (or perhaps "This *can't* be happening to me!") and "My life will never be the same" and "Whose fault is this?" These are only some of the thoughts and questions that start spinning through the minds of people affected by this diagnosis.

Remember that I described therapy as "providing good information, objective feedback, and solid encouragement in a supportive, confidential setting." It becomes apparent, doesn't it, that this kind of psychological treatment will be necessary and helpful? Some research suggests that the first year after a diagnosis of bipolar disorder is a crucial time for people with the illness. The education, support, and encouragement that psychotherapy provides are vital in making treatment successful in the long term.

Another traumatic event that people with bipolar disorder face all too frequently is relapse. The management of bipolar disorder is still far from perfect, and despite everyone's best efforts, relapse can and does occur. Many people feel like they're "back to square one" when this happens. They may blame themselves or their medication or their doctor; they may become angry, disappointed, discouraged, and confused about what to do next. Again, counseling helps the person put things back into perspective, get over the setback, and move on.

PSYCHOTHERAPY FOR BIPOLAR DISORDER

There are many different approaches to helping people with bipolar disorder through psychotherapy.

Cognitive Behavioral Therapy (CBT)

As we saw in earlier chapters, the available pharmaceutical treatments for the depressed phase of bipolar disorder are less than perfect by a long shot. The mood stabilizers are not entirely as effective as antidepressants for some people, and antidepressant medications carry the risk of precipitating mania or accelerating the frequency of cycles. But psychotherapy has a proven track record in helping with depression. Importantly, it has no chance of precipitating mania or of accelerating the course of bipolar disorder.

In the 1960s, Dr. Aaron Beck and his colleagues developed a theory of depression and psychotherapeutic treatment for it called *cognitive behavioral therapy*, or CBT for short. There is more research to support CBT for depression than most other types of therapy. It has a proven track record of helping with symptoms of depression. Some studies—though not others—have found CBT to be as effective as antidepressant medication for some people with depression.

The theory of cognitive behavioral therapy maintains that people with chronic or frequent depression have developed a distorted view of themselves and the world. It proposes that these individuals have adopted patterns of thinking and reacting to challenges that actually perpetuate their problems. This emphasis on thinking, or *cognition*, lends the theory and the therapy its name. As we saw in chapter 1, people with depression tend to (1) think negatively about themselves, (2) interpret their experiences negatively, and (3) have a pessimistic view of the future. Cognitive theory calls this the *cognitive triad*. The theory further proposes that all this negative thinking causes a person to develop a repertoire of mental habits called *schemas* or *negative automatic thoughts*. These are habits that spring into action and reinforce negative thinking.

This means that in situations that can be interpreted in many different ways, both positive and negative, people go for the negative out of habit. They don't seek alternative positive explanations. This, in turn, sometimes causes them to do things that reinforce negative thinking, and the vicious cycle repeats itself.

Here are several negative schemas that people with bipolar disorder are prone to:

Negative: "I got manic even though I was taking my lithium. It doesn't matter what I do. What's the use?"

Realistic: "Relapses occur even with medication. It might have been much worse and lasted much longer if I hadn't been on medication. Perhaps this new medication will be more effective for me."

Negative: "Everyone will avoid me when I go back to work. No one wants to work with a mentally ill person."

Realistic: "Some people might avoid me at work, perhaps many at first. But when they see that I'm the same old me, they'll come around. And those who don't are people I don't want as friends anyway."

There are cognitive therapy techniques specifically focused on bipolar disorder. Part of the treatment deals with the negative automatic thoughts that interfere with treatment by medication. For example, if a person with bipolar disorder is troubled by the negative automatic thought "Taking mood-stabilizing medication is a sign of personal weakness" every time they take a dose of lithium, they might be more likely to skip doses or stop taking the medication altogether. Cognitive therapy works on the psychological barriers to proper treatment by replacing automatic negative thoughts with realistic ones.

Specialized CBT

There are several subtypes of CBT that deserve mention.

Dialectical behavioral therapy (DBT) is a form of CBT for the treatment of borderline personality. This complex psychiatric problem involves difficulty modulating (or controlling) emotions, as well as other problems. In addition to working on distorted thinking, people receiving DBT also focus on modulating their emotional reactions to stressful situations.

Other goals of DBT include defusing intensifying emotional situations, coping with uncomfortable feelings, and preparing for crises. A group of researchers at the University of Pittsburgh developed and tested a form of DBT specially tailored to adolescents with bipolar disorder. They compared this form of DBT to treatment as usual in a small group of adolescents with bipolar disorder. The volunteers were "relatively ill youth who had early illness onset, psychiatric hospitalizations, and poor functioning." At the end of the study, the adolescents in the DBT group "demonstrated significantly less severe depressive symptoms . . . and were nearly three times more likely to demonstrate improvement in suicidal ideation."

Mindfulness-based cognitive therapy (MBCT) is another variation of CBT. As its name suggests, it teaches the individual to become more aware of thinking patterns and emotional states by noticing and observing mood fluctuations and changes in symptoms. The focus is to observe these changes in a nonjudgmental way and to respond in a calm, preplanned manner. Meditation is also a component. In a study on twenty-three volunteers with bipolar disorder treated for eight weeks, MBCT reduced anxiety and enhanced mindfulness. It also improved emotional regulation and a cognitive skill called *executive functioning*, which, loosely defined, means "thinking before acting." The volunteers in this study also had a functional magnetic resonance imaging (MRI) scan before and after their treatment. This is a specialized brain imaging technique that shows activity levels in different parts of the brain. Compared to before their course of MBCT, the scans of the volunteers with bipolar disorder showed a return toward normal in areas of the brain known to be underactive in people with depression. Of note, these volunteers were either in a normal mood state or having only mild symptoms, indicating that even these relatively well people with bipolar disorder benefited from MBCT.

Group Psychotherapy

Psychotherapy can be very effective in a group setting. The worry I often hear expressed by patients about group therapy is that they don't want to "sit around listening to other people's problems." But no group therapist worth their salt will let the group deteriorate into a "pity party." Instead, they will guide the group members onto the track of learning from and helping solve one another's problems—not just venting about them. An excellent way to become a better problem solver is to see how other people solve or fail to solve their problems. By observing and reacting objectively to another person's issues, group members learn how to think more objectively and less emotionally about their own.

In traditional group psychotherapy, people with a variety of problems are in the group. In the treatment of bipolar disorder, however, *homogeneous* groups (composed exclusively of people with bipolar disorder) have been studied. These more specialized groups are more effective. Several studies show that people with bipolar disorder who attend group therapy have fewer relapses and improved productivity at work or school. One research study found that the shared aspect of the problems discussed in the sessions seems to be integral to the therapeutic experience. People with bipolar disorder who are in groups with other people with bipolar disorder report that practical advice from others about living with the illness is extremely helpful. Their understanding of the disorder, of how it affects their relationships and self-attitudes, is enhanced. They perceive the guidance they receive from other group members as invaluable.

This aspect of group therapy—sharing and learning from one another—is the basis of another type of "therapy," one that doesn't require a therapist: peer support groups. We shall discuss this helping format in the next part of this book.

I've already mentioned a kind of therapy called psychoeducation. This type of treatment is especially suited to a group setting. A *psychoeducational group* combines more traditional group therapy with an instructional or classroom approach. It often includes reading materials and discussion questions about bipolar disorder. These may include information about symptoms, the warning signs of relapse, and how to better communicate with family members, employers, and coworkers regarding the illness, among other topics. A presentation of facts about the illness or techniques for dealing with it becomes a takeoff point for discussing the individual's experiences and using new knowledge to feel better and function more effectively. A study of people who were "minimally symptomatic" compared how effective attending a psychoeducational group was compared to individual therapy. The researchers found that each treatment improved the individuals' functional level and residual symptoms—and the group treatment was much less expensive. For this and other reasons, this approach is gaining favor. Numerous studies have shown psychoeducation to be a valuable adjunct to other treatment approaches to bipolar disorder.

"Traditional" Psychodynamic Psychotherapy

I hope I haven't given you the impression that traditional psychotherapy isn't helpful for people with bipolar disorder. Quite the contrary. Kay Redfield Jamison has written:

At this point in my existence, I cannot imagine leading a normal life without both taking lithium and having had the benefits of psychotherapy. Lithium prevents my seductive but disastrous highs, diminishes my depressions . . . and makes psychotherapy possible. But, ineffably, psychotherapy *heals*. It makes some sense of the confusion, reins in the terrifying thoughts and feelings, returns some control and hope and possibility of learning from it all.

So far in this chapter, I've talked about treatments that focus on helping people deal with specific issues related to an episode of illness. These include the stresses of diagnosis, hospitalization, and reintegration back into their jobs. I've discussed CBT and its variations, which focus on chronic or smoldering depressive symptoms that medication alone doesn't seem to entirely take care of, as well as being more alert to emotional states and triggers.

Psychodynamic psychotherapy doesn't focus on symptoms or a particular set of problems. The goals of this type of therapy are more profound: self-understanding, self-acceptance, and personal growth. The patient and the therapist will, of course, talk about symptoms like sadness and anxiety as well. But traditional psychotherapy emphasizes exploring the *meaning* of symptoms and the development of self-awareness and maturity. This process may take place over an extended period of months or even years.

When would this type of psychotherapy be recommended to a person with bipolar disorder? For what kinds of problems would it be helpful? Basically, for the same problems that people without bipolar disorder go to therapists for: dealing with psychological traumas and setbacks—both past and present—that cause feelings of sadness, anger, or anxiety. Psychodynamic therapy can focus on anything that disrupts a person's ability to be happy in relationships, effective at work, carefree in play, or confident about making decisions about the future. If that sounds like a tall order, it is. That is why psychotherapists often study and train in their profession for as many years as physicians do. That is why people are sometimes in therapy for months or even for years at a time. That is why psychotherapy is such an intense, powerful experi-

ence, and the therapeutic relationship between patient and therapist a unique one.

People with bipolar disorder have often had more than their
share of setbacks and psychological traumas—both past and present. Because it is a genetic illness, people with bipolar disorder
have often had difficult, even traumatic, childhoods. Perhaps a
parent was afflicted with the illness. Maybe the parent could not
or would not receive proper treatment. The child may have suffered disruptions to family life, periods of poverty or homeless-
ness, or even physical or emotional abuse. This type of therapy
can be enormously beneficial in helping people face and work
through their difficult pasts. It can help them let go of the anger,
resentment, and fear that often come from these experiences and
move on with their lives.

PSYCHOTHERAPY IN BIPOLAR DISORDER: IS IT REALLY NECESSARY?

**Many research studies have demonstrated that psychother-
apy helps individuals with bipolar disorder stay well and
improve their functional level.**

There are many reasons why people with bipolar disorder may be
reluctant to get into therapy. Some of them have made an uneasy
peace with taking medication for a psychiatric illness but see
going to psychotherapy as confirmation of the "mental" aspect
of their "mental illness." But if you think about it, the treatment
of even the most "medical" of medical illnesses—heart disease,
say, or a ruptured lumbar disk—usually requires nonmedical interventions. Sometimes these interventions turn out to be just as
important as the doctor's pharmaceutical or surgical treatments.
The recovering heart surgery patient wouldn't ignore the physician's recommendation for a cardiac-hardening exercise program.
Would anyone have an operation for lumbar disk problems and
skip the physical therapy sessions afterward? I don't think so.

We know that chronic psychological stresses make various physical illnesses—asthma, high blood pressure, and irritable bowel syndrome, to name just a few—more difficult to treat. Psychological stresses will make mood-disorder symptoms more difficult to control as well.

The fact that a person has bipolar disorder can make everyday life decisions seem complex and overwhelming. There is no better way of dealing with these sorts of anxieties and apprehensions than psychotherapy. I remember a young woman who came to see me for a routine medication-monitoring appointment when working in the hectic medication clinic of a community mental health center. In this busy clinical setting, patients were scheduled every twenty minutes. "I've been dating a man for several months now, and I think he might ask me to marry him," she told me. She looked worried. "I haven't told him about my illness. I don't know what to tell him. How do you think I should handle this?" I stared at her helplessly for a moment and panicked just a little when I heard the nurse slipping the next patient's chart into the bin outside the interviewing-room door. I hope I didn't sound as rushed as I felt when I tried to convince her that the situation raised many complex issues. Adequately dealing with the questions of how, when, where, why, and with whom she discussed her diagnosis was going to need much more than one—or a dozen—twenty-minute appointments with me.

I doubt very much that this was the first time this young woman had been confused about telling someone about her diagnosis. Perhaps she muddled through other situations at work, at church, or in her neighborhood, maybe saying nothing about her diagnosis because of feelings of shame or maybe blurting out too much about herself and then feeling vulnerable and exposed. Perhaps being diagnosed with bipolar disorder reactivated feelings she had struggled with in childhood or adolescence about being teased for being too fat or too skinny—or perhaps, more likely in an individual with bipolar disorder, for being "hyper" or "weird." I was sure that since we had discussed the fact that bipolar disorder is a genetic illness, a marriage proposal must have raised questions in her mind about having children who might be affected by the disorder. How had the diagnosis affected her identity as a potential parent, as a woman? Or perhaps none of these issues needed to be explored, but instead other, completely different ones. Well, all of these issues are what good old-fashioned once-a-week "How do you feel about that?" psychotherapy is all about.

A 2016 review paper analyzed more than thirty clinical trials of psychotherapeutic interventions for bipolar disorder, including psychoeducation groups, CBT, DBT, MBCT, and several others. The authors' happy conclusion was that "psychotherapy interventions for the treatment of bipolar disorder have substantial evidence for efficacy."

There are many forms of psychotherapy because some work better than others for particular people. It may take several tries to find the best match for an individual patient. People with bipolar disorder owe it to themselves to take advantage of the unique healing powers of these wonderful therapeutic techniques.

Key Takeaways

❖ *Psychotherapy should be considered an integral part of the treatment of bipolar disorder, as crucial for people with this illness as physical therapy is for a patient who has suffered a heart attack or stroke.*

❖ *A large body of clinical research has established that many forms of psychotherapy, including several specially developed to treat bipolar disorder, effectively reduce symptoms and promote improved functioning.*

PART III

Getting Better and Staying Well: What You Can Do

❖There are millions of people living with bipolar disorder today. Many are living healthy, happy, and productive lives, but many others are not. This part of the book is intended to help you maximize your chances of getting into and staying in the first category and staying out of the second. People with bipolar disorder need to take charge of their treatment.

Chapter 8 tells you how. If you're looking for a simple list of dos and don'ts, I'm afraid you will be disappointed. In this chapter, I discuss the most important reason why some people with bipolar disorder do poorly: a lack of commitment to treatment.

❖The third leg of the three-legged stool of the treatment of bipolar disorder is a set of lifestyle changes that reduce physical and psychological stress, known as *de*-stabilizers, for this stress-sensitive illness.

Chapter 9 is all about a set of good habits that lead to better outcomes, a collection of habits that I call *mood hygiene*. Regularizing sleep is perhaps the most important, but you can do many other things to control symptoms and prevent relapses.

❖**Despite everyone's very best efforts, emergencies arise. Be prepared!**

Chapter 10 offers some principles for dealing with emergencies and highlights the types of situations that people with bipolar disorder and their families often fail to prepare for. We're always tempted to put off thinking about and planning for things we hope won't happen. But it is essential not to give in to this temptation. I explain here how easy it is to be prepared for emergencies.

❖**Bipolar disorder doesn't only affect the individual diagnosed with the illness.**

Inevitably, family and friends are affected in countless ways by this disease, both directly and indirectly. Chapter 11, "Family Matters," addresses this aspect of the illness. I talk about what family members can do—and, just as important, what family members cannot and should not try to do—to help their loved one who has bipolar disorder.

CHAPTER 8

Living with Bipolar Disorder

At present, there is no cure for bipolar disorder, only treatment and management. It is a relentless illness that, left untreated, will inevitably and repeatedly return to torment its sufferers. The only way to keep it at bay is for the person who has it to be relentless as well—relentless about getting needed treatment and sticking to it.

ACCEPTANCE AND COMMITMENT

The first steps towards successful treatment are to accept the diagnosis and make a commitment to treatment.

Human beings have an almost unlimited capacity to explain away the obvious. People who don't want to confront serious physical illnesses can ignore and rationalize even the most alarming symptoms—for example, the middle-aged man with a history of high blood pressure who doesn't pay attention to his repeated episodes of chest pain ("Oh, it's just heartburn; must have been something I ate") or the woman who feels a lump in her breast and tells herself, "It's probably just a cyst, I'm sure it will go away." Facing a possibly life-threatening illness is perhaps the most frightening experience we can encounter. Small wonder that we sometimes put ourselves through some impressive mental gymnastics to avoid the confrontation.

When there are no *physical* signs of illness, no pains or lumps or dizzy spells, it may be easier to convince oneself that the symptoms of illness are something else. People not infrequently ask whether they need to continue on a mood stabilizer after a manic episode has resolved. They may say, "After all, I was under a lot

Will There Ever Be a *Cure* for Bipolar Disorder?

Until we have a much better understanding of the causes of bipolar disorder, it's hard to imagine what a cure might look like, if by *cure*, one means a one-time intervention that resolves symptoms and eliminates any chance of recurrence. However, at the beginning of the twentieth century, the idea of a cure for cancer seemed like an impossible dream. Yet today, many forms of cancer are eminently curable. In 2011, a cure for hepatitis C became available. Gene therapies are under development for various immunological diseases and sickle cell anemia.

A cure becomes a much more difficult thing to imagine when an illness is essentially a developmental problem like schizophrenia appears to be. And one of the daunting problems with developing a cure for bipolar disorder is that there seem to be many "broken" pieces to fix. There are probably dozens of genetic errors that add up, probably in many different combinations, to cause a person to develop the illness.

So while the best we can do right now is to *control* the symptoms, a recent scientific development may lead to dramatic improvements in treatment. This development is a technique by which any cells from an adult can be transformed into stem cells, which are then coaxed to develop into neurons. In the future, a technician might take a few skin cells from a patient (like a dermatologist might take a "punch" biopsy to check a suspicious mole) and then use those skin cells to grow neurons in the lab. Those neurons could then be tested to see exactly what functions have gone awry, and treatments would be selected based on that information. Such techniques are already in use for cancer treatment and hold great promise for treating other illnesses.

Even more exciting is the possibility of using a patient's stem cells to treat the illness directly. Such interventions to treat neurological diseases like Parkinson's are already in development. Stem cells appear to be able to find their way to damaged areas of the brain and help rebuild what's been lost in these illnesses. By the time you read this, a clinical trial under the leadership of Dr. Jair Soares at the UTHealth McGovern Medical School in Houston will be under way, involving infusing stem cells into people with bipolar depression.*

So although we can't speak of a cure just yet, exciting changes in the treatment of bipolar disorder may be just over the horizon.

* Information about this and other clinical trials for bipolar disorder is available at https://clinicaltrials.gov.

of stress, and I hadn't slept for weeks. Maybe I just need to take it easy." As we'll see, stress can indeed play a role in precipitating an episode of a mood disorder, *but it's not the cause*. Stress doesn't give people mania or send them into a major depression unless they have bipolar disorder. Neither does drinking too much or sleep deprivation or the loss of a job or the end of a love affair, or the hundred other things that you can convince yourself of to explain your symptoms.

People with bipolar disorder can go through years of denial and anger about their illness. I have seen patients repeatedly stop taking medication and drop out of treatment because of this. Instead of taking the condition seriously, they explain their repeated hospital admissions, shattered relationships, and ruined finances in all sorts of ways. "My wife has it in for me. She put me in the hospital again." "If my boss wouldn't put so much pressure on me, this wouldn't happen." "I think you need to recheck my thyroid; I know that's the real problem." Or, in its simplest form: "I don't need this medicine because I'm not crazy."

If you have been diagnosed with bipolar disorder and you have read to this point in the book, you may have already gotten past a great deal of this understandable denial and anger. This is a significant accomplishment—it signals a turning point in your journey towards recovery.

In bipolar disorder, the individual ultimately determines how well *any* treatment will work—because it is the *individual* who puts treatment recommendations into action. It is the individual who will determine whether they take *every* dose of medication, or just ninety percent of the doses, or fifty percent, or even less. The individual will determine whether the blood for their lithium or valproate blood-level test is drawn exactly twelve hours after the last dose or whether they get to the lab after ten or fifteen hours, throwing the results and the doctor's calculations off by ten or twenty percent. The individual will determine how many appointments they keep with the doctor and the therapist and how many they miss—and how many are shorter than scheduled because of tardiness. It's so easy to let your guard down, let treatment lapse in little ways, and convince yourself that missing a dose of medication here or there, having that second beer, ignoring a string of sleepless nights isn't really important. To do so is to turn away from rather than confront this disease, and often the turning away springs from ambivalence about the need for treatment—from *less than complete acceptance of the diagnosis*. To not accept this illness, to not confront it, puts the treatment's success in jeopardy, because in bipolar disorder—perhaps more than in any other serious illness—it is the individual who administers the treatment most of the time.

Making a commitment to treatment means (1) being active, not passive, in formulating a treatment plan with your providers;

Getting Better and Staying Well: The Essentials

- Make the decision that you will do whatever it takes to take control of this illness; otherwise, it *will* take control of you.

- Be *active*, not passive, in collaborating with your treatment providers.

  - *Prepare* for your appointments. What is your goal for today's appointment?

  - Write down your observations and any questions ahead of time and bring them to the appointment.

  - Ask your prescriber to give you any changes in the treatment plan *in writing*. Don't rely on memory. Hospitals and clinics can usually provide you with an *after-visit summary* with a medication list, blood tests ordered, and so forth. Ask for it!

- Take charge of your treatment—by taking medications as directed, getting blood tests done as ordered, and keeping appointments (and being on time!)

(2) taking charge of treatment implementation 100 percent of the time; and (3) making the decision that you will do everything possible to take control of this illness rather than be controlled by it.

WHY RELAPSE PREVENTION IS SO IMPORTANT

Emil Kraepelin, the German psychiatrist who literally wrote the book on bipolar disorder in the early twentieth century, cared for his patients at a time when there were no effective treatments for the illness he called "manic-depression." He was able to observe how the illness ran its course in individuals when nothing could be done to alter its progression with medications. Kraepelin noticed that early in the course of his patients' illnesses, mood episodes often appeared to be triggered by some stressful event in their lives: "In especial, the attacks begin not infrequently after the illness or death of near relatives. . . . Among other circumstances there are occasionally mentioned quarrels with neighbors or relatives . . . excitement about infidelity, financial difficulties. . . ." Kraepelin noticed, however, that later in the course of the illness, attacks occurred "wholly without external influences." That is, they happened without any trigger.

The accuracy of these observations has been borne out in later studies. Observational studies of people with bipolar disorder have shown that:

• Early in the course of their illness, mood episodes occur usually after some trigger in the environment. Later in life, they tend to arise without any identifiable trigger.

• Individuals can experience an acceleration in their illness as they age, with episodes occurring more and more frequently as time goes on.

• More mood episodes make people *more* sensitive to stress and *more* likely to relapse than they might otherwise be.

Researchers followed fifty-two people with bipolar disorder for two years and kept track of the number of episodes they experienced. They found that people with more prior episodes were more sensitive to stresses. People with a higher number of prior episodes were more likely to relapse under stress and they relapsed more quickly.

But the converse appears to be true as well: as time in remission gets longer, people appear to tolerate stress better and this helps

"The Second Year on Lithium Is Better Than the First"

That adage is one that a professor of mine was quite fond of saying—both to patients and to his trainees and students. Over the years, I've come to agree with him. But our Johns Hopkins colleague Dr. Kay Redfield Jamison, an internationally recognized expert on bipolar disorder who also suffers from it, did him one better.

Several years ago, I was leading a seminar for psychiatry residents at Johns Hopkins on the treatment of bipolar disorder with lithium, and we were lucky enough to have Professor Jamison drop by and join us. As we were finishing up, I repeated my colleague's maxim—"The second year on lithium is better than the first"—to the trainees. Smiling mischievously, Dr. Jamison added, "That's right . . . and the *twenty*-second year on lithium is really terrific!" Her point, amply demonstrated by research, was that more extended periods of mood stability confer resilience on people with bipolar disorder. They lessen the probability that stresses will trigger an episode.

them to stay well. Longer periods of mood stability appear to *protect* people with bipolar disorder from relapsing under stress. Longer remissions lessen the probability that stresses will trigger an episode. This fact gives people an opportunity to significantly improve their course of illness. *The key to doing well over the long term is to prevent relapses.*

Several studies have demonstrated that preventing mood episodes improves long-term outcomes in bipolar disorder. Treatment intervention during the first ten years after diagnosis appears to be the most important factor in success. The prevention of manic episodes is especially critical.

Working hard to stay well, especially in the first years after diagnosis, will make it easier to stay well over the longer term. Put another way, stability leads to more stability. And there should be no doubt in your mind at this point that the most effective relapse-prevention tool is medication.

People with bipolar disorder should make peace with the idea of taking medication every day for the foreseeable future. That is an especially hard thing to do in this disease. The symptoms and the need for medication often start when people are in their twenties or even younger. At this age, very few of their peers must bother with medication. They may think that the only people who take medication are "old people" and "sick people." It's difficult for a young, physically healthy person who's feeling well to take medication every day.

Each individual needs to work out for themselves a method for making sure that they take every single dose of every medication. Pharmacies sell a variety of clever devices to help make this happen. There are boxes that hold a whole week's worth of medication in little compartments, one for every dose, so that the answer to "Did I take my dose this morning?" is always clear and certain: if the little compartment is empty, the dose was taken. Even if you take only one medication every day, this simple tool is worth your investment of money and time. Smartphone and smartwatch "medication tracker" apps are available, too.

Why Do People Stop Taking Medication?

In my very first year as a psychiatric resident, a patient with severe mania was being admitted to the unit where I was working. I was in the nurses' station, writing progress notes on another patient, when I heard the unit secretary hang up the phone and announce to the staff in the area, "That was the ER. Becky [not her real name] is coming back!"

"Oh my," said one of the nurses. "She's only been out for a month this time; usually, it's more like three months." It seemed I was the only one on the unit who didn't know Becky.

A few minutes later, Becky's old records arrived at the unit—all five volumes of them (this was in the pre-electronic medical record days of paper records). They showed that Becky had a highly lithium-responsive case of bipolar I disorder. However, she had stopped taking her lithium again and again and had needed rehospitalization again and again. The pattern had gone on for years. As the clinical picture became clear, I remember thinking, "How hard can it be to take a few lithium capsules every day? Why would anyone choose to live like this?" In the years that followed, I learned that, as is so often the case in psychiatry, the answer is complicated.

In a study from the early days of lithium therapy in the United States (1979), researchers interviewed people about their reasons for stopping lithium. They said they were "bothered by the idea that moods are controlled by medication" or "by the idea of [having a] chronic illness."

More recent studies have confirmed that people's

attitudes toward medication are important factors in why they stop taking it. These factors include fear of becoming dependent on medication, shame about taking psychiatric medication, and seeing all medications as inherently unnatural or unhealthy. Interestingly, problems with side effects are consistently low on the list. Recent studies have again confirmed that discomfort with having one's mood "controlled" by medication is an important factor.

It's perhaps not a surprise, then, that the most effective treatment interventions for improving adherence to medication recommendations are *psychoeducational programs*. These are programs, usually in a group setting, that provide information on bipolar disorder and its treatment. Psychoeducational programs help people identify stressors and triggers, avoid substance use, and recognize the early signs of relapse.

As for the idea that medication is "controlling" one's moods, I tell patients that the much more accurate way of thinking about this is to recognize that *medication gives back your ability to control and modulate emotions*, rather than allowing bipolar disorder symptoms to hijack them. Without medication, the illness's abnormal moods take control *away* from you.

K. R. Jamison, R. H. Gerner, and F. K. Goodwin, "Patient and Physician Attitudes Toward Lithium: Relationship to Compliance," *Archives of General Psychiatry* 36, no. 8 (1979): 866–69. https://doi.org/10.1001/archpsyc.1979.01780080040011.

Emilie Leclerc, Rodrigo B. Mansur, and Elisa Brietzke, "Determinants of Adherence to Treatment in Bipolar Disorder: A Comprehensive Review," *Journal of Affective Disorders* 149, no. 1–3 (2013): 247–52. https://doi.org/10.1016/j.jad.2013.01.036.

Ask your treating physician whether your medication can be taken just once a day, or twice, rather than three times a day. Studies have shown that when a medication must be taken three times rather than two times a day, the number of doses a person actually takes drops off significantly. Ask about controlled-release forms of medications; they often make it possible to eliminate midday doses. These are the most difficult ones to fit into a busy life.

The body of evidence showing that medication is a major factor in preventing relapse cannot be argued with; it is simply overwhelming. But there is another important reason why preventing relapse is so important, particularly in people taking lithium. There is significant evidence that people who stop taking lithium run the risk of lithium not being as effective for them when they restart.

A study published in 2017 found that over a quarter of people who stopped taking lithium for bipolar I and II disorder did not respond to it as well when they restarted it. This was especially true of people who relapsed while they were not taking it. More than one in ten of these people no longer responded to lithium at all and in another thirteen percent, lithium was only somewhat effective. This problem has been called *lithium-discontinuation-induced refractoriness*. It is not known whether this is true of other medications for bipolar disorder.

ALCOHOL AND DRUGS ARE MOOD DESTABILIZERS

In study after study, it has been shown that individuals with bipolar disorder who misuse alcohol and drugs do poorly compared with those who do not. However, substance misuse is not uncommon among people with bipolar disorder. A 2016 analysis of over 65,000 individuals with bipolar disorder from seventy-eight different studies found that over one-third of men and nearly one in twenty women with bipolar disorder also met the diagnostic criteria for an addiction diagnosis.

Alcohol and drug abuse appear to cause episodes of abnormal

mood in people with bipolar disorder. Perhaps they trigger episodes in people who are vulnerable to the disorder because of
genetic factors. Several studies have shown that people with bipolar disorder who have a substance-abuse disorder have a stormier
course to their mood disorder than people who do not abuse alcohol or drugs. On average, "dual-diagnosis" people (people with
a diagnosis of bipolar disorder and addiction) develop symptoms
of their bipolar disorder at a younger age. In some studies, they
have been shown to have more frequent hospitalizations. This has
been interpreted to indicate that substance abuse may worsen the
course of bipolar disorder, perhaps because of some direct effect
on the brain caused by repeated use of drugs and alcohol.

All abused substances (including alcohol) appear to work by
stimulating the "reward" centers of the brain. You have probably heard that laboratory animals will push a lever that delivers
an electrical stimulus to these brain regions and ignore the lever
that delivers food to their cage until they're practically dead from
hunger. When a similar lever device is used to deliver an intravenous dose of alcohol or another drug to laboratory animals,
the substances that animals self-administer in this way are almost
exactly the same ones that humans abuse and become addicted to:
opioids, cocaine, and certain stimulants and tranquilizers. These
drugs all work the same way: they disrupt the normal operation
of the brain's "feel-good" circuitry.

Now, you don't need to be a psychiatrist to realize that people
with bipolar disorder already have enough problems with the
"feel-good" circuits of the brain and that further mucking things
up with "recreational" drugs is a terrible idea. There is some evidence to suggest that intoxicating substances actively interfere
with the therapeutic effects of the medications used to treat mood
disorders.

My patients often ask me, "Can I have an occasional glass
of wine with dinner?" Although I'm hard-pressed to forbid my
patients ever to drink, it's clear that when it comes to alcohol, less
is better.

Cannabis: Use at Your Own (Considerable) Risk

Although the research literature on the issue is not extensive, what literature there is indicates that people with mood disorders should avoid using cannabis.

One of the difficulties with research in this area is that *Cannabis sativa*, the marijuana plant, contains hundreds of psychoactive substances whose effects vary widely. Making things more complicated is that different *C. sativa* strains have varying amounts of these compounds.

The two main psychoactive cannabis compounds (*cannabinoids*) are delta-9-tetrahydrocannabinol (THC) and cannabidiol (CBD). THC is responsible for the cannabis "high" as well as its adverse effects, which include anxiety, panic, paranoia, and psychosis, while CBD has antianxiety and other therapeutic effects. Most recreational cannabis consists of higher THC and lower CBD potency, meaning that using cannabis recreationally should be thought of as using THC. This fact likely explains why the preponderance of the research evidence indicates that cannabis has predominantly adverse effects on mental health. The link between cannabis and schizophrenia is now well established: cannabis doubles the risk of developing schizophrenia and, in people with schizophrenia, causes them to have more severe symptoms, higher rates of relapse, more extended hospitalizations, and a poorer quality of life. Ironically, however, pure CBD preparations are being investigated for their *antipsychotic* effects.

(continued)

The research on cannabis's effects on people with mood disorders is less extensive but also strongly indicates that recreational marijuana use is harmful to these individuals. Studies of depression also show an increased risk of being diagnosed with major depressive disorder, earlier age of onset, and worse symptom progression. Studies in individuals with bipolar disorder indicate that cannabis contributes to longer mood episodes, increased mood cycling, lower remission rates, increased suicide risk, and lower recovery.

There are also studies in people with mood disorders that found no evidence of harm—clearly, more research needs to be done. However, a recent review paper that summarized dozens of studies concluded, "The current literature indicates that there are more harmful consequences compared to benefits associated with long-term cannabis use in bipolar disorder symptomatology and disease progression."[*]

*D. J. E. Lowe, J. D. Sasiadek, A. S. Coles, and T. P. George, "Cannabis and Mental Illness: A Review," *European Archives of Psychiatry and Clinical Neuroscience* 269, no. 1 (2019): 107–20. https://doi.org/10.1007/s00406-018 -0970-7.

USE OR ABUSE? DO I HAVE A PROBLEM?

The overuse of alcohol and drugs can best be understood as a problem *behavior*. A behavior becomes a problem when the individual engages in it despite negative, even self-destructive consequences. A person has a substance-misuse problem if they continue to use an intoxicating substance despite the physical, psychological, or social problems that it is causing or making worse. Substance misuse is not defined by how much or how often a person uses it.

Loss of control and *continued use despite negative consequences* define substance abuse.

When bipolar disorder and a substance-misuse problem coexist, they both need treatment. Getting proper treatment for the mood disorder will make the substance-abuse problem easier to treat, but it cannot be assumed that a substance-misuse problem will simply go away when a coexisting mood disorder is treated.

Signs of Alcoholism

Many medical and professional organizations endorse the CAGE questionnaire to identify problem drinking:

1. Have you ever felt you should **C**ut down on your drinking?

2. Have people **A**nnoyed you by criticizing your drinking?

3. Have you ever felt bad or **G**uilty about your drinking?

4. Have you ever had a drink first thing in the morning to steady your nerves or get rid of a hangover (an **E**ye-opener)?

One *yes* suggests a possible alcohol problem. More than one *yes* means that an alcohol problem is highly likely.

J. A. Ewing, "Detecting Alcoholism: The CAGE Questionnaire," *Journal of the American Medical Association* 252, no. 14 (1984): 1905–7. https://doi .org/10.1001/jama.1984.03350140051025.

Key Takeaways

❖ *The first steps towards successful treatment are to accept the diagnosis and make a commitment to treatment.*

❖ *Relapse prevention is one of the most important goals of treatment for bipolar disorder. Repeated episodes make additional ones more likely, and stability begets stability.*

❖ *Alcohol and drugs are powerful destabilizers of mood for people with bipolar disorder.*

CHAPTER 9

The Elements of Mood Hygiene

Mood hygiene **is a set of practices and habits that promote better control of mood symptoms. These lifestyle changes are the third leg of the three-legged stool of bipolar disorder treatment.**

"HYGIENE": AN UNDERUSED WORD IN PSYCHIATRY

Hygiene is a word that we probably don't use as often as we should in psychiatry, and we certainly don't use it as much as we used to. Hygeia was the Greek goddess of health, the daughter—or in some versions of the story, the wife—of Asclepius, the god of medicine. Hygiene, or hygienics, is the science of *the establishment and maintenance of health* as opposed to the treatment of disease. It is concerned with conditions and practices that promote health. The hygienic conditions and practices we think of today usually relate to cleanliness, but the word has a much broader meaning. At the beginning of the twentieth century, institutions such as the Johns Hopkins University School of Hygiene and Public Health (now the Bloomberg School of Public Health) and the London University School of Hygiene and Tropical Medicine were founded to study methods for *preventing* disease. They aim to improve the health of whole communities. The National Committee for Mental Hygiene was founded in 1909 by former asylum inmate Clifford Beers (who probably had bipolar disorder). Now called Mental Health America, this organization promotes emotional health and well-being and lobbies for better and more readily available treatment for psychiatric illnesses.

Several areas of research on bipolar disorder demonstrate that preventive measures improve symptom control. Things like lifestyle regularity and stress management make a big difference. Mood hygiene is the third leg of the three-legged stool of bipolar disorder treatment. Unlike the other two, however, this aspect of treatment is entirely in the hands of the individual.

THE PRIMACY OF SLEEP

The most critical element of mood hygiene is close attention to getting a good night's sleep—every night!

Paying attention to our body's natural rhythms is a very important—perhaps the *most* critical—component of mood hygiene. Sleep deprivation can precipitate mania in people with bipolar disorder. Even one night of total sleep deprivation can destabilize mood to the point where hospitalization is needed.

To understand the relationship between sleep and mood, you need to understand a little about how the body's sleep system works. Chronobiology (from *khronos*, the Greek word for "time") is the science of bodily rhythms and biological clocks. It turns out that nearly every living thing has an internal biological clock. Even organisms as simple as bacteria turn out to have an internal time-keeping mechanism. We humans are no different.

An important concept in chronobiology is that of *circadian rhythms*. The term comes from the Latin words *circa*, meaning "around," and *diem*, meaning "day." It refers to rhythms in the body that have an approximately twenty-four-hour cycle, like the day-night cycle. Many bodily functions follow a circadian rhythm. Our body temperature cycles daily, with the lowest body temperature occurring at about four a.m. and the highest at around seven p.m. Blood pressure drops while we are asleep and jumps up at about seven a.m.

Research has shown that when there is a disruption to our internal clock, it negatively affects our mood. English researchers demonstrated this in an experiment that has become a classic in the field of chronobiology. For this experiment, fourteen healthy young men and women volunteered to live in experimental living quarters for several weeks and follow a thirty-hour sleep-wake cycle instead of the usual twenty-four-hour schedule. Their "day" consisted of twenty hours of wakefulness and ten hours of sleep. Every several hours, while awake, they took a ten-minute battery of psychological tests and rated their mood. The researchers found that the volunteers' internal clocks went in and out of synchronization with their artificially imposed sleep-wake cycle. Furthermore, the more out of synchronization the volunteers were, the worse their mood became. And remember, these were *healthy* volunteers. The experiment showed that when our sleep wake cycle and our internal clock are out of sync, it has a strong *negative* effect on our mood. Bottom line: even people who do not suffer from mood disorders have mood symptoms when the sleep-wake cycle is disrupted. For those with bipolar disorder, the consequences can be downright dangerous.

There have been numerous reports of individuals with bipolar disorder having manic episodes after transatlantic flights or after sleep deprivation caused by medical emergencies or family crises.

But it doesn't take a transatlantic flight to cause problems for people with bipolar disorder. Even relatively minor disruptions can be destabilizing. When researchers followed a subgroup of about 200 subjects from the STEP-BD study for a year and evaluated their sleep and mood, an unmistakable pattern emerged. Volunteers who had fewer total hours of sleep in the week before their appointment had more manic symptoms. Volunteers whose sleep patterns varied widely from one night to the next had more depressive symptoms. There is, of course, a "chicken and egg" question here. Did sleep disruption cause the mood symptoms in these volunteers, or did a mood change cause the sleep problems? Given what we know about total sleep deprivation triggering mania in people with bipolar disorder and sleep cycle disruption causing mood changes in healthy volunteers, I think it's not a stretch to conclude that the former is the case: sleep problems *cause* mood problems in people with bipolar disorder.

Just as people with diabetes who want to do well need to be careful about their diet, people with bipolar disorder need to be

How to Take Care of Your Sleep: Sleep Hygiene

- Set a daily schedule for getting up and going to bed. If possible, do this every day.

- Eliminate screens in the late evening.

- Avoid caffeine: drink "half-caf" coffee and no-caffeine soft drinks. If you can't do without, make a "no caffeine after noon" rule for yourself.

- Don't drink alcohol in the evening. Alcohol is good at inducing sleepiness but has the opposite effect when it comes to maintaining sleep. As the alcohol level in the bloodstream drops during the night, the brain wakes up—and you'll wake up, too!

- Avoid large meals late in the evening.

- Don't smoke before bedtime. Nicotine is a stimulant.

- Reserve the bedroom for sleep and intimacy and avoid activities that promote wakefulness in the bedroom. Don't eat or watch TV in bed, even during the day.

- Regular exercise is beneficial for a good night's sleep.

careful about their sleep. An essential part of mood hygiene is *sleep hygiene*.

Getting a better night's sleep means taking active steps to protect your biological clock from disruptions in the environment. Our sleep-wake cycle is set every morning by exposure to bright light upon awakening. What follows from this fact are the two most important principles of good sleep hygiene: (1) keeping to a regular schedule by going to bed and getting up the same time every day, and (2) making sure to limit exposure to light at the wrong times. In this regard, the most common culprits are the ubiquitous screens of twenty-first-century life: TV screens, computer screens, phone and tablet screens. Computer, phone, and tablet screens are especially problematic because they are enriched with blue wavelengths. As far as your biological clock is concerned, playing a computer game at ten p.m. is like walking outside on a bright sunny morning with a lovely blue sky. You are essentially giving your brain a strong signal that it's time to wake up—not to get ready for bed!

STRESS MANAGEMENT

Psychological stress is a significant trigger for mood episodes. It's also the risk factor that you can do the most to mitigate.

Next on the list of mood-hygiene practices is *stress and conflict management*. Most of us have little control over when and how stress and conflict come into our lives. But we can learn how to manage stress and conflict better—and here I'll put in another plug for counseling and therapy. This is because I am talking about serious, *vigorous* attention to whatever ongoing sources of serious stress there may be. Primary relationship and marital conflicts, job and career problems, and chronic financial or legal problems are good examples. Immediately after a diagnosis of bipolar disorder may not be the time to deal with ongoing and chronic problems of these sorts. But several months later, after mood symptoms have been under good control for a while, it is a good time for some very serious stocktaking. Professional help can be highly beneficial.

By *stocktaking,* I do not mean some process that can be described in a few paragraphs or distilled into the kinds of "helpful hints" and "dos and don'ts" lists that you might find in a magazine article. Instead, I mean *serious examination and fundamental change.* This may involve changing jobs or even careers, selling a house that you can't afford, or declaring bankruptcy instead of struggling with an austerity budget. It might mean postponing or reconsidering marriage (or divorce) or not going back to school. A person who has had a heart attack must do some serious investigation and hard thinking before taking a job as a high-level manager of a big company. A person with bipolar disorder needs to go through the same process before making big decisions. This is one reason why therapy and counseling are such a vital part of the treatment of bipolar disorder. Being able to get objective feedback and help in working out these important decisions is invaluable.

STRUCTURING YOUR LIFE

Having a structured life is often a foreign concept to people with bipolar disorder. They have often lived unpredictable lives because of unpredictable mood fluctuations. Once mood fluctuations are better controlled on medication, it becomes possible to put more structure in place. As I've already mentioned, structuring the sleep-wake schedule is critical. But a structured life is a less stressful life. Structure and schedules eliminate the anxiety that comes with worrying whether you will have time to do what needs to be done.

Make regular days and perhaps even standard times for whatever your everyday chores are, whether that means housekeeping, paying the bills, mowing the lawn—whatever. If you're a student, make regular study times, and no cramming or all-nighters!

Regular exercise has been shown to benefit sleep and has many other benefits. It helps to stabilize blood pressure, for example, most likely because it reduces the level of the stress hormone *cortisol* in the body. As you'll read in part IV, "What Causes Bipolar Disorder?," cortisol turns out to be highly detrimental to brain functioning. Put simply, regular exercise is not only good for your muscles, bones, and heart; it's good for your brain. *Schedule* your daily walk and your Monday-Wednesday-Friday swim or visit to the gym. Don't exercise only when you "have the time" or "feel like it." Make it part of your regular schedule, not a luxury.

Don't allow yourself to procrastinate. Putting things off until the last moment invariably increases stress levels. Waiting until the eleventh hour to work on your income tax return and then staying up late, tanked up on coffee and searching for receipts and W-2 forms, is not something people with bipolar disorder should let happen to themselves. It's no fun for anybody, but for the individual with bipolar disorder, it's downright dangerous. File your taxes early, renew your driver's license early, get your car inspected early—you get the idea. Eliminate procrastination as a way of dealing with things, and you've gone a long way toward eliminating a lot of stress. This advice holds for putting off dealing with interpersonal problems, too. Smoldering tensions in a relationship or chronic conflicts with a coworker, a neighbor, or a landlord—these are chronic stresses that will inevitably take their toll on *anyone's* mental health. They can exact a higher price on the individual with a mood disorder. Don't put off dealing with these problems. If you don't know how to approach them, get the professional help you need, whether that means consulting a counselor or a therapist or an attorney.

Alcohol? As I've already said, *the less, the better.*

Psychological stress, sleep deprivation, lack of exercise, alcohol and drugs, and even an unhealthy diet are all environmental factors that raise cortisol levels in the bloodstream. And as I've already mentioned, the stress hormone cortisol has a directly damaging effect on neurons, especially the neurons in a brain structure called the *hippocampus*. This is an area of the brain that, as you'll see later, is at the center of mood control. Whatever you can do to keep cortisol levels down will make it easier for your medication to work to keep you well.

Some people find it helpful to keep a record of their moods, a *mood chart*. This can be a journal or diary if you're so inclined, but more straightforward and less time-consuming techniques can work just as well. If you need to keep an appointment calendar anyway, it's a simple matter to record your mood daily using a numerical scale. Clinicians commonly ask patients to rate their mood on a one to ten scale, with "one" being the most depressed they've ever felt and "ten" being the best mood they've ever had. "Five" is a normal, neutral, everyday mood. If one to ten seems too confining, use a scale of 1 to 100. It's important to rate your mood at the same time every day to control for diurnal (daily) mood variations. Simply record your mood ratings every day by jotting down a number in your appointment book, recording it in your computer time-management program, or marking it on a calendar you keep on your bedside table. One of the first things I ask my patients to do when they're having trouble with persistent mood cycling is to keep a more detailed mood chart that also captures changes in their sleep pattern, menstrual cycle, levels of anxiety, and medication changes. A well-kept mood diary can be an invaluable aid to your treatment team.

A quick internet search is all it takes to find any number of blank mood charts you can easily print out. You will also find several websites that allow you to set up an account and track your symptoms online. Mood-tracker apps for smartphones are available, too. Keeping this kind of record will provide you and your clinical team with invaluable information that can help show what medications are or are not working. It can help determine whether there is a premenstrual or seasonal component to mood changes. It can also detect evolving depressive or hypomanic episodes earlier, when it's easier to intervene.

All of this is much easier said than done for people with bipolar disorder. Regularizing your life in these ways may seem entirely foreign and strange, not to mention boring. If throughout your life you've learned to wait for the good moods to get things done and just put off thinking about things during the inevitable return of the bad ones, such planning and regularity won't come easily. But a growing body of research supports the notion that external regulators like regular sleep and activity schedules help with mood stability. Recognizing this and putting it into action is what mood hygiene is all about.

MAKING CHANGES: YOU CAN DO IT!

After reading the last chapter and getting this far in this one, you may be wondering whether *you* have some bad habits that need to change. Night-owl computer gaming? Cocktails *and* wine with dinner most nights? A couch-potato lifestyle? So how does behavioral change work?

The essential prerequisite for making a change in any problem behavior is accepting the need to change—that is, recognizing that the behavior is causing problems, is out of control, and needs to be given up. This is often the most challenging step. Unless the person overcomes denial ("This isn't a problem; I can stop any time I want to") and accepts their need to change, the change process can't even get started.

One way to conceptualize the process of recognizing this need to change behavior is the *transtheoretical model of behavioral change*, more commonly called the "stages of change" model. Initially developed to define the thought patterns and process of behavioral change in smoking cessation, this model proposes that individuals who successfully change an unhealthy behavior pass through several stages in the process of change in a highly predictable way (figure 9.1).

The first phase is called the pre-contemplative stage. In this

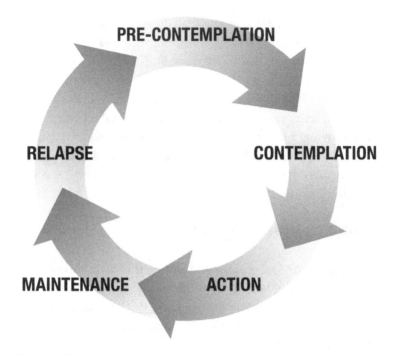

Figure 9.1. The stages of change in the transtheoretical model. *Source: Illustration by Jenna Macfarlane.*

phase, individuals simply don't consider that they may have a problem. They see no reason for making a change because they have little or no appreciation of the negative consequences or even danger of their behavior.

The next phase is known as the contemplative stage. At this point, individuals begin to see that their behavior has at least some negative consequences—to themselves and their health or their loved ones. They are beginning to think there might be some advantages to stopping the behavior and may even take some steps to investigate what that might entail. They have made no commitment to stop, but they are at least somewhat open to the possibility of stopping. This is a critical part of the cycle because it is a pivotal place to intervene. People can be stuck here for some time: they may fear the difficulty of stopping, feel uncertain about putting together a plan, or just be "waiting for the right time." This is sometimes as far as a person gets in the process of change. It can be a difficult time in their life; they now see the negative results of their actions, but are still powerless to stop.

The third phase is known as the action stage. Individuals take steps to implement a plan to stop their negative behavior. This is also a crucial stage in the process—if the individual can't tolerate the loss of the behavior's positive effects, they may quickly give up on their plan and move back to the contemplation phase. During the action stage, individuals need support, empathy, and strong encouragement to keep on track and continue in treatment.

If individuals' actions lead to the cessation of the behavior, they enter the maintenance stage. At this stage, they continue to abstain from negative behaviors. They have coping mechanisms and support in place to keep doing so. As with the action phase, individuals may need a great deal of support to remain committed. This can be particularly important as their situation improves and the negative consequences of the behavior recede. It is easy to see how seductive thoughts like "just one more time" or "I can handle it now" can sneak in.

Most mental-health professionals are well-equipped to help people who want to change a problematic behavior, whether it's something as relatively minor as overreliance on procrastination as a way of coping with a too-busy life or something as serious as problem-drinking or even drug addiction.

The first step is admitting that there might be a problem. This is often the most challenging step. People with problem behaviors engage in them because doing so benefits them in some way. This may seem counterintuitive, and most people turn out to be quite surprised by the number of *positive* aspects of a problem behavior they hadn't realized existed.

What are the good things about drinking too much? Drinking alcohol makes you feel good. It is an expected part of many social situations. It decreases anxiety, increases self-confidence, and boosts one's mood, at least initially. In large amounts, it dead-

The Stages of Behavioral Change

The *transtheoretical* model of behavior change proposes that people pass through characteristic and predictable phases on the way to changing a self-defeating behavior, whether it is weight loss, cigarette smoking, alcoholism, or "cutting" behaviors. People make behavioral changes in stages, moving clockwise through the cycle from *pre-contemplative* (not accepting the need to change) to *maintenance* (maintaining the behavioral change). Many slip backward (counterclockwise in the cycle) on their way to recovery. Many suffer a full relapse, moving from maintenance to the pre-contemplative phase and needing to go through the cycle another time, even multiple times, before achieving success.

It's important to emphasize here that whether *others* think that negatives outweigh positives is not important. Only the affected individual's judgment in this matter can lead them to change.

- Pre-contemplation stage:
    - "I don't have a problem."
    - "I can stop any time I want to, but I don't need to or want to."

- Contemplation stage:
    - "Maybe this is a problem, but I'm not ready to change."

> - Action stage:
>   - "I have a problem. I definitely need to stop doing this and start developing a plan to do so."
> - Maintenance stage:
>   - "I need to be vigilant; it would be so easy to slip up and be right back where I started!"

ens the psychic pain of depression to some extent—at least for a few hours. However, we know that alcohol and other intoxicating substances worsen depression when used regularly. It's easy to see how an individual can continue a behavior if they judge that the negative consequences do not outweigh its benefits.

Start by making a list of the good things about and the detrimental aspects of the behavior you want to change. What are attractive things about the behavior you want to change, and what are the negative consequences of not changing? If you get stuck, ask your therapist for help doing so. Then develop an action plan and get the support you need to stick with it.

Key Takeaways

❖ *Mood hygiene is the third leg of the three-legged stool of treating bipolar disorder. It's all about healthy habits.*

❖ *Establish regular sleep habits: retire to bed and get up at the same time every day.*

❖ *Avoid sleep-disrupting habits: cut down on caffeine and avoid electronic tablets, smartphones, and other screens in the late evening.*

❖ *Structure and schedule your days: make time for exercise—and relaxation.*

❖ *Keep a mood chart or use a mood app on your smartphone.*

❖ *Take stock of sources of stress in your life.*

   • *Job problems? Relationship problems? Worries about the stigma of a psychiatric diagnosis? Therapy, therapy, therapy!*

   • *Don't procrastinate—it's a recipe for worry.*

CHAPTER 10

Preparing for Emergencies

Although emergency situations are nearly unavoidable for people with bipolar disorder, "emergency" doesn't need to mean "crisis" — if you're prepared.

The decisions we are forced to make in a crisis are frequently not the decisions we would have made under other circumstances. When an emergency arises for which we are unprepared, we usually have to improvise a response as we go along. In this chapter, I identify several potential emergencies that the individual with bipolar disorder and their family may face, and discuss how to prepare for and deal with them. One of the best ways to prepare for an emergency is to have a crisis plan ready beforehand.

Because we have such effective treatments available for bipolar disorder, we sometimes forget that it is a potentially lethal illness. And when you are dealing with a disease that can become life-threatening, the last thing you want is an improvised response to an emergency.

People usually enjoy making plans—vacation plans, wedding plans, retirement plans. Planning for a psychiatric emergency is much less enjoyable but, unfortunately, much more important. Unlike vacation plans, these are plans that no one would be disappointed about not getting to use. But if you do need them, odds are you'll be very glad you made them.

KNOW WHOM TO CALL FOR HELP

I've always thought that the people who can handle almost anything are those who know when they need help and whom to
call for it. People with bipolar disorder owe it to themselves to be
under the care of a psychiatrist who is familiar with their symptoms and the course of their illness. That means establishing yourself with a new physician when you move to a new community
or if any other factor, such as the retirement of your psychiatrist,
leaves you "uncovered." Changes in insurance plans sometimes
force a change in psychiatrists. Don't put off making an appointment to get established as a new patient. Because administrative
hassles and delays can prolong the time it takes for records to be
transferred from one office to another, ask your providers for a
copy of your records or a letter of introduction that you can take
to your new doctor at the first appointment.

Don't hesitate to ask the psychiatrist how their practice is cov-
ered after hours. How easy is it to get a routine office appointment?
Are appointment slots set aside so that urgent appointments are
available within a day or two? Every psychiatrist or mental health
clinic should have some means of seeing patients within twen-
ty-four hours in case of an actual emergency.

Be sure you know how to contact the psychiatrist or their office
at any time of the day or night and what arrangements are in place
to handle emergencies. Does the psychiatrist always see their
patients for emergencies, or does everyone in the practice take
emergency on-call duty on a rotating basis? This type of "on-call"
system, though not ideal, is often standard; it means that you may
well not see your regular doctor in an acute emergency. Are you
prepared for such an arrangement in order to be under the care of
a psychiatrist who comes highly recommended?

What hospitals does your prescriber or their practice have a
relationship with? Do they admit to the hospital you prefer? To
the hospital where your insurance covers inpatient psychiatric
treatment?

If the answers to these questions are not satisfactory, consider your options. Ask your family doctor, family members, friends, or members of your support group for recommendations.

SAFETY ISSUES

The most dangerous emergency for people with bipolar disorder, and one that frequently leads to hospitalization, is the development of suicidal thoughts and behaviors. Bipolar disorder has the highest rate of suicide of all psychiatric conditions, and the risk of suicide is approximately twenty to thirty times that of the general population.

It may seem obvious to say that the most effective way of minimizing the risk of suicide in bipolar disorder is relapse prevention. But if I had said *"relapse* prevention is *suicide* prevention" in chapter 8, you might have thought I was just being dramatic. Do not *ever* lose sight of the fact that bipolar disorder is a potentially fatal disease: relapse prevention *is* suicide prevention.

The emergence of self-destructive thoughts and impulses is frightening both to the person with bipolar disorder and to those around them. The tremendous stigma and disgrace that have been associated with suicide for centuries still make people reluctant to discuss these thoughts when they occur. That context and notions such as "only crazy people kill themselves" complicate what is really a much simpler clinical issue: suicidal thinking is a serious symptom of this illness, which must be evaluated quickly by a professional and managed swiftly and effectively. People can be intensely ashamed of suicidal thoughts and believe that the development of self-destructive impulses is a kind of failure. Of course it is not a failing in any way; it is a symptom of an illness. It is important to understand the development of suicidal feelings in a person with bipolar disorder as a dangerous symptom of a serious illness, as dangerous as the onset of chest pains in a person with heart troubles. When they occur, it's not a time to wonder about what they mean. *It's time to call for help.* And like chest pains in a person with heart troubles, suicidal feelings in a person with a mood disorder are often a reason for hospitalization.

Psychiatric hospitalization can be perceived as a terrible failure. Again, the clinical perspective tells us otherwise. Although we have become much better at treating bipolar disorder, our treatment methods are by no means perfect. Sometimes, despite everyone's best efforts, relapses occur and serious symptoms like suicidal feelings emerge and require hospitalization. Such an occurrence is not time for self-blame or questions like "What did I do wrong?" Rather, it's time for healing.

Remember that the word we often used in the past for psychiatric hospitals was *asylum*, a term defined as "a place offering protection and safety." Individuals whose will has been temporarily seized by this terrible illness and who are on the verge of terrible and desperate action deserve a place of protection and safety. No apologies are *ever* necessary, and no reproach is ever justified.

One more important point about safety: individuals with bipolar disorder should not have firearms in the home. There are numerous scientific studies showing that this increases the chances of a violent death occurring in that home, either by suicide or by homicide. Where an illness whose symptoms can include suicidal depression and heightened irritability with loss of inhibitions is concerned, there is never, *ever* any justification whatsoever for having a firearm of any type in the home. Period.

One more reminder: bipolar disorder can raise issues of personal safety. These issues need to be anticipated, discussed, planned for, and promptly addressed if and when they arise. Because family members are often a crucial part of dealing with these emergencies, I'll discuss their role further in the next chapter.

Key Takeaways

❖ *Have an emergency plan. Decisions made in crisis mode are usually not the best ones.*

❖ *Thoroughly research your insurance plan to understand your options.*

❖ *Do not have firearms in the home.*

CHAPTER 11

Family Matters

The challenges of living with bipolar disorder are not limited to those who have the disease. Family and friends face challenges as well. It's intensely painful to see a loved one suffer from the desperate bleakness of major depression and just as painful and frightening to see them in the fierce grip of mania. As in any illness, the role of the family includes support, understanding, and encouragement of the person who is ill. The first step in providing this kind of support is understanding some essential facts about the illness.

RECOGNIZING SYMPTOMS

Never forget that the person with bipolar disorder does not have any control over their mood state. Those of us who do not suffer from a mood disorder sometimes expect those who do to be able to exert the same control over their emotions and behavior that we ourselves can. When we sense that we are letting our emotions get the better of us and want to subdue them, we tell ourselves things like "Snap out of it," "Get hold of yourself," and "Pull yourself out of it." We often think that self-control is a sign of maturity and self-discipline. We may believe that people who don't control their emotions are immature, lazy, self-indulgent, or foolish. But you can only exert self-control if the control mechanisms are working properly. In people with mood disorders, they are not.

People with mood disorders cannot "snap out of it," however

much they would like to (and it's important to remember that they *desperately* want to be able to). Telling a person with depression things like "Pull yourself out of it" is cruel. Worse yet, it may reinforce the feelings of worthlessness, guilt, and failure that the person is experiencing, which are symptoms of the illness. Telling a person with mania to "Slow down and get a hold of yourself" is simply wishful thinking; that person is like a tractor trailer careening down a mountain highway with no brakes.

The first challenge facing family and friends is to change the way they look at behaviors that might be symptoms of the illness. These may be behaviors like not wanting to get out of bed, being irritable and short-tempered, being "hyper" and reckless, or being overly critical and pessimistic. One natural reaction to these sorts of behaviors and attitudes is to get angry. We often regard the person who behaves in such a way as lazy, mean, or immature, and then we may criticize them. In a person with bipolar disorder, criticism almost always makes things worse: it reinforces the feelings of worthlessness and failure when that person is depressed. And it alienates and angers the person with hypomania or mania.

This is a hard lesson to learn. Don't always take behaviors and statements at face value. Before you react, learn to ask yourself, "Could this be a symptom?" Little children come out with "I hate you" when they are angry at their parents. But good parents know that it's just the anger of the moment talking; what the child says doesn't reflect their deeper feelings. People with mania will say, "I hate you" too, and it's the illness talking—an illness that has hijacked the person's emotions. The person with depression will say, "It's hopeless; I don't want your help." Again, it's the illness and not your loved one rejecting your concern.

I'm now going to make things really difficult by warning against the other extreme: interpreting *every* strong emotion in a person with a mood disorder as a symptom. This other extreme is just as important to guard against. I have seen many couples in which one partner has bipolar disorder, and the healthy partner wields the diagnosis as a weapon to emotionally subdue the other.

A clinical vignette about Vicky (not an actual patient) will help illustrate this point.

"Vicky's medication needs an adjustment. I'm sure of it," said Peter. Vicky stared down at the floor angrily as Peter, her husband, went on: "She won't give up on this crazy idea about going back to college."

I winced a little at Peter's use of the word *crazy*, a word that can make a person with a psychiatric illness feel like they've just been slapped in the face. I made a mental note to bring it to his attention later, but to do so now might make it look as though I were "taking sides."

"Peter," I said, "I'd like to hear from Vicky about this. She's been doing well for over two years now; I think it may be time to have a serious discussion about her idea."

Vicky looked up and spoke: "I was six months away from graduating college when I got sick the first time. I've called some other schools about re-enrolling, and I could get my degree with only a year of study at any one of them."

Vicky was in her mid-thirties, an intense, vibrant woman who, I suspected, was probably brilliant as well. Peter had been transferred to the area by his company a month after Vicky had gotten out of the hospital. It had taken three hospitalizations for her to be correctly diagnosed as having bipolar disorder—after nearly ten years of roller-coaster moods. She had been treated for a depressive disorder, for a personality disorder, even for schizophrenia before she started on the correct medication and had a big turnaround. She had done so well, in fact, that I had seen her only half a dozen times over the past two years. About half the time, her husband came along to her appointments. Every couple of months, I noticed a book review she had written in the local newspaper. On one visit, she mentioned working on a biography of John F. Kennedy. Going back to university seemed well within her capabilities.

Peter sighed and spoke up again: "It makes me really nervous to see her up late at night, looking at college entrance requirements on the internet. We've gotten dozens of university brochures through the mail that she's called or written for. I'm afraid she's getting manic, and I just can't go through that again."

Vicky's eyes flashed. She drew in her breath, then slowly released it. "Peter's not used to me being this confident and energized about anything. We've only been married for four years, and for nearly two of those, I was more or less depressed. This is me, not mania." Her voice became just the slightest bit louder. "But he's treating me like a child, an incompetent." She looked over at her husband. "A lunatic, right? I'm finally getting back to my goals and career after ten years, and what did you call it? 'Crazy,' wasn't it?"

Now it was Peter's turn to look angry. "You see, Doctor? Do you see what I mean, how angry she gets? She's not usually like this. Before we came here today, she—"

"Oh, God, stop it," Vicky said quietly, through clenched teeth. Tears were flowing now.

"OK, you two, let's cool down for a moment," I said. I could sense that this was a continuation of a power struggle between Peter and Vicky that had probably been going on for weeks, maybe even months. But I also had the sense that Vicky was assessing herself accurately and that Peter was overreacting. Vicky was not being carried away by her feelings—not at the moment; if anything, she was showing a lot of restraint. Peter *was* treating her like a child. "Vicky," I said, "perhaps Peter doesn't understand your reasons for wanting to go back to college."

"I admit it might seem like a waste of time," she said. "But that degree means a lot to me. I was devastated when I had to withdraw from the university. I felt like a complete failure. Maybe I just need to prove to myself that I can do it. That I'm not . . ." She hesitated before spitting it out: "not crazy."

Peter was calmer, too. "It's not that we can't afford it," he said. "I just worry that it will be too much for her, that she'll get sick again. And she gets so angry when we talk about it; she seems obsessed with this idea. That's not normal, is it?"

"I don't think trying to decide how much obsessiveness is normal or abnormal is going to help us here, Peter," I said. "The problem it seems to me is that Vicky is investing a lot of time and emotional energy in a project that you don't think is worthwhile."

"That's right," Peter said decisively.

"But I think it's worthwhile," Vicky said. "Just because I have a psychiatric illness doesn't invalidate me as a person. It doesn't mean I need someone to make all my decisions for me."

"Honey, I'm just trying to help you, to protect you—"

Vicky snapped back, "I don't want to be protected, I want to have a real life."

"Wait a minute, wait a minute," I said. "I think we were getting somewhere. Let's go back to Vicky's reasons for wanting to go back to school."

This struggle between Peter and Vicky illustrates a common problem that can come up in families in which an individual has been diagnosed with a bipolar illness. It's possible to jump to the conclusion that everything the ill person does that might be foolish or risky is a symptom of their illness, even to the point of hauling the person into the psychiatrist's office for a "medication adjustment" every time they disagree with their spouse, partner, or parents. As with Peter and Vicky, a vicious cycle can take over: some bold idea or enthusiasm, or even plain old foolishness or stubbornness, is labeled as "getting manic" and stirs up feelings of anger and resentment in the person with the diagnosis. When the person with bipolar disorder expresses angry feelings, they seem to confirm the family's suspicion that the person is "getting sick again." More criticism ensues, followed by more anger, and so on.

"They're getting sick again" sometimes becomes a self-fulfilling prophecy, triggering so much anger and emotional stress that a relapse *does* occur. Perhaps the person with the illness stops taking medication out of frustration and shame: "Why bother staying well if they *always* treat me as if I were sick?"

So how does one walk this fine line between not taking every feeling and behavior at face value in a person with bipolar disorder, on the one hand, and not invalidating real feelings by calling them symptoms, on the other? I think communication is the key: honest and open communication. Ask the person with the illness about their moods; make observations about their behaviors; express concerns in a caring, supportive way. Go along with your family member to doctor's appointments, and share your observations and concerns during the visit in the family member's presence. Above all, do not call the therapist or psychiatrist and say, "I don't want my [husband, wife, son, daughter] to know that I called you, but I think it's important to tell you that . . ." There's nothing more infuriating or demeaning than to have someone reporting on you behind your back.

But it's also possible to err on the side of not being involved enough in treatment for fear of being a tattletale. Don't assume that the clinicians will notice the same things you've noticed about changes in moods or behaviors. One of the most valuable ways a family member can help is to provide a clear, undistorted view of the situation to the clinical team treating the illness. In my experience, family members are frequently the first to pick up on subtle changes in behaviors and attitudes that signal the beginning of a relapse. Over the years, I have often seen patients in the clinic or even in the emergency room who reassured me that they felt fine. And since their behavior and mood seemed normal, I sent them on their way with a note in the chart that they were doing well. Many a time, I've then received a panicked phone call from a spouse or other relative a few hours later: "Didn't he tell you that he's lost ten pounds?" ". . . that she hasn't slept in three nights?" ". . . that he got fired from his job?" Contrary to popular belief, psychiatrists cannot read minds! Become involved with treatment, and communicate your concerns openly, sincerely, and supportively. Almost anything that might otherwise seem intrusive can be forgiven.

Remember that your goal is to have your family member trust you when they feel most vulnerable and fragile. They are already dealing with feelings of deep shame, failure, and loss of control related to having a psychiatric illness. Be supportive and, yes, be constructively critical when criticism is warranted. But above all, be open, honest, and sincere.

INVOLUNTARY TREATMENT

In every community, there are laws and procedures to safeguard individuals who cannot care for themselves. Laws that allow the removal of children from the care of parents who are abusing them are the most obvious example. Another set of laws enables individuals to be treated for psychiatric illnesses against their will in certain circumstances. One of the most challenging things a person might be called on to do for a family member with bipolar disorder is to initiate involuntary treatment or commitment. But given the power of this illness (especially bipolar I) to cloud one's judgment and create dangerous situations, there is sometimes no choice but to force the treatment issue in this way. It is always a last resort, but it can be lifesaving.

Commitment laws can vary by jurisdiction, and local procedures can vary from community to community. Therefore, I can't provide a step-by-step approach here, only general principles. But in my experience, it's not the procedures that confuse people, it's the general principles, and so I think a brief discussion is worthwhile.

Laws and legal procedures governing the provision of psychiatric treatment—or any kind of medical treatment, for that matter—against a person's stated wishes are based on the knowledge that the symptoms of an illness can cloud an individual's judgment. When this happens, they often do not make the same decisions about treatment that they would make otherwise. The delirious motor-vehicle-accident victim who has suffered massive blood loss may moan "I want to go home" as they lose consciousness on the stretcher. But the ambulance crew will ignore such a statement and proceed to do whatever they have to do to save the person's life. They have presumed that if the person were thinking clearly, they would not make such a request.

Similar principles underlie psychiatric commitment laws: treatment is given to people against their will if clouded judgment prevents them from making good decisions about their treatment. Individuals with depression may feel so hopeless that they believe the treatment has no chance of helping. Thinking processes in mania can be so disorganized and scattered that seeking out and cooperating with treatment is impossible. In either case, there are mechanisms to get needed treatment for people whose psychiatric symptoms blind them to the need for it.

MORE ON SAFETY

Never forget that bipolar disorder can occasionally precipitate truly dangerous behavior. Violence is often a difficult subject to discuss. This is because the idea is deeply embedded in us from an early age that violence is primitive and uncivilized and represents a kind of failure or breakdown in character. Of course, we recognize that the person in the grip of psychiatric illness is not violent because of some personal failing. Perhaps because of this, there is sometimes hesitation in admitting that there is a need for a proper response to a situation getting out of control: some threat of violence toward oneself or others.

I've already talked a bit about suicidal thinking. It bears repeating that people with bipolar disorder are at much higher risk for suicidal behavior than the general population. Family members cannot and should not be expected to take the place of psychiatric professionals in evaluating suicide risk. However, they should have some familiarity with the issue. Again, people who are starting to have suicidal thoughts are often intensely ashamed of them. They will often hint about "feeling desperate," about "not being able to go on," but they may not verbalize actual self-destructive thoughts. It's important not to ignore these statements but rather to clarify them. Don't be afraid to ask, "Are you having thoughts of hurting yourself?" People are usually relieved to talk about these feelings and get them out into the open. But they may need permission and support to do so.

Remember that the recovery period from a depressive episode can be a time of especially high risk for suicidal behavior. People who have been immobilized by depression sometimes develop a higher risk for hurting themselves as they begin to get better and their energy level and ability to act improves. People with mixed symptoms—depressed mood and agitated, restless, hyperactive behavior—may also be at higher risk of self-harm. There is some evidence that mixed or dysphoric mania is the most dangerous mood state in this regard.

Another factor that increases the risk of suicide is substance abuse, especially alcohol abuse. Alcohol not only worsens a person's mood, it also lowers a person's inhibitions. People will do things when they are drunk that they wouldn't do otherwise. Increased use of alcohol increases the risk of suicidal behaviors. It is a worrisome development that needs to be confronted and acted on.

The development of serious suicidal risk calls for action. Have an emergency plan and be prepared to use it. Don't hesitate to invoke involuntary commitment procedures if you are really worried and the person is disputing the need for an evaluation.

A less frequent but real risk of violence is the violence toward others that can occur in mania. Friends and family members should not hesitate to call for help if they feel imminently threatened.

Many communities have teams of mental health professionals who can respond to behavioral health emergencies. They have specialized training in de-escalating situations involving people with psychiatric problems. Sometimes, these crisis intervention teams are part of the local police department. The team consists of specially trained police officers accompanied by a clinical social worker or other mental health professional.

In 1992 the city of Houston, Texas, established an entire police department division specializing in mental health issues. Houston trains not only patrol officers but also call center dispatchers and jail personnel to recognize and respond appropriately to situations involving people with mental illness.

In an ideal world, a phone call for help with an imminently violent person with bipolar disorder would result in a rapid response from a team of various professionals trained in crisis intervention who are accustomed to dealing with psychiatrically ill individuals. They would be knowledgeable about safe physical restraint techniques and familiar with psychiatric emergency services in the community. They would have the capability to transport the person quickly and safely to the appropriate health care facility for proper treatment. Unfortunately, we do not live in an ideal world, and many communities do not provide these kinds of services. Tragedies have resulted when inadequately trained police officers have overreacted in confrontations with aggressively agitated people with psychiatric illnesses. Such tragedies highlight the importance of being familiar with the full range of available emergency services in your community and developing emergency plans with your or your loved one's treatment team.

GETTING SUPPORT

Family members need to recognize their own need for support, encouragement, and understanding in dealing with this illness. Mental-health professionals go home every day and leave their work of dealing with psychiatric illnesses behind, an option that family members often do not have. It can be exhausting to live with a person with hypomania and frustrating to deal with a person with serious depression day after day. The changes in mood and the unpredictability of someone with bipolar disorder intrude into home life and can be a source of severe stress in relationships, straining them to the breaking point.

Perhaps the most difficult challenge is that posed by a family member with bipolar disorder who is resistant to obtaining treatment. The most remarkable learning experience that medical students and interns have is with their first patient who repeatedly refuses to continue with a treatment that will keep them well and out of the hospital. It takes a while and more real-world experience before these students understand that making peace with an illness and with the idea of staying in treatment is much more complicated than healthy people realize.

But the more brutal lesson is that there is no way anyone can *force* a person to take responsibility for their treatment. Unless the patient commits to doing so, no amount of love, sympathy, cajoling, or even threatening can make someone take this step. Even family members who understand this at some level may feel guilty, inadequate, and angry at times when dealing with this situation. These are completely normal feelings. Family members should not be ashamed of experiencing frustration and anger; rather, they can seek help with handling these emotions.

Even when the individual does take responsibility and is trying to stay well, relapses can occur. Family members might then wonder what *they* did wrong. Did I put too much pressure on them? Could I have been more supportive? Why didn't I notice the symptoms coming on sooner and get them to the doctor? Swirling questions, mounting regrets, rounds of *if only*: guilt, frustration, and anger.

On the other side of this issue is another set of questions: How much understanding and support for the bipolar person might be too much? What is protective, and what is overprotective? Should you call your loved one's boss with excuses for why they aren't at work? Should you pay off credit card debts from hypomanic spending sprees caused by dropping out of treatment? What actions constitute helping a sick person, and what actions are helping a person to be sick? These are thorny, complex questions that have no easy answers.

For all these reasons, it's vital that family members go along with the bipolar individual to support groups—and go to support groups themselves even if the person will not go—and consider getting counseling or therapy for themselves to deal with the stresses caused by this illness. Comprehensive programs for the treatment of people with bipolar disorder are increasingly emphasizing family involvement.

Like many other chronic illnesses, bipolar disorder afflicts one but affects many in the family. It's important that all those affected get the help, support, and encouragement they need.

Key Takeaways

❖ *Family members should familiarize themselves with the signs of a developing mood episode. That being said, people with bipolar disorder are allowed to have normal feelings.*

❖ *Become familiar with involuntary treatment procedures and community resources in your area, and have an emergency plan at the ready, especially if the diagnosis is bipolar I disorder and there is a history of suicidal behaviors.*

❖ *Family members need support too!*

PART IV

What Causes Bipolar Disorder?

❖Since the late 1990s, neuroscientists have made a great deal of progress in understanding the causes of bipolar disorder. This progress has already led to better treatments. Understanding even a little about this illness's causes will help you understand the reasons behind treatment recommendations.

"What causes this illness?" "How does lithium work?" "What is this medication doing in my brain?" For more years than I care to remember, when my patients asked me these questions, I could only answer, "No one really knows." That was the sad truth. All this mysteriousness naturally made some people reluctant to take medications and others to look askance at their providers' urgent counseling to avoid sleep deprivation and learn to manage stress better (which sounded like clichés anyway).

Since the turn of the twenty-first century, answers to these questions have started to emerge. Neuroscientists have a better understanding of the effects of lithium and other drugs on brain functioning. It's possible to visualize how the condition alters the brain structure of people with bipolar disorder and how stress affects the brain.

With this knowledge, the treatments and other recommendations begin to make sense. I think it's a lot easier to put treatment recommendations into practice if you understand how and why they work. That's why I wrote this section of the book.

The fine details of brain functioning are complicated and subtle, which is why I'm skipping over most of them. But many of the basics are not at all difficult to grasp. Yes, there are some big words in this section—science is science, after all—but they are easily explained. And no specialized knowledge is needed to understand the concepts in any of the pages that follow.

And yes, this part of the book can be considered optional reading. However, understanding a little of the science behind what you've been reading so far will make it much easier to see why the recommendations of the previous part are so important. It will help you feel better about marshaling the effort needed to put them into practice. I urge you to persevere!

CHAPTER 12

Bipolar Disorder in the Brain

■ By investigating the effects of lithium on the brain, neuroscientists have discovered that lithium has a *protective* effect on brain cells that may underlie its efficacy in treating bipolar disorder. This breakthrough has opened up new ways to investigate the causes of bipolar disorder.

■ Brain imaging studies have revealed that there are several brain networks involved in emotional regulation. People with bipolar disorder appear to have communication disturbances between the brain areas that make up these networks.

LITHIUM AND THE BRAIN

Although John Cade described the therapeutic effects of lithium for all phases of bipolar disorder in 1949—effects stumbled upon purely by chance, if you remember—it was many decades before anyone figured out just what lithium was doing in the brain that might be helping. As medications go, lithium is uniquely effective in treating bipolar disorder, so it quickly became apparent that figuring out what lithium does in the brain would lead to understanding what causes bipolar disorder. But before we get to that, we need to talk about stress.

HOW THE BODY HANDLES STRESS

The most dramatic bodily response to stress is the familiar "fight or flight" response. Suppose you are hiking along the Appalachian Trail and suddenly encounter a bear twice your size. In that situation, some dramatic physical changes will take place in the body. These changes either prepare you to face combat with the creature ("fight") or, perhaps more likely, to run as fast and as far as you can ("flight"). There is a hormonally triggered flood of energy-containing glucose, fat molecules, and proteins into your bloodstream; your heart rate and blood pressure go up to get these energy molecules to the muscles as quickly as possible. Your breathing becomes faster and deeper to provide the oxygen needed to turn those energy molecules into power. At the same time, the body systems that are *not* involved in fighting or fleeing shift down. Digestion slows, cellular growth and tissue repair grind to a halt, and even the immune system temporarily goes into hibernation. All of this is just what a physical emergency requires. However, if this hyperactive physiology goes on for too long, bad things begin to happen in the brain. These negative effects have been well documented in stress experiments in mice and rats. Let's briefly explore these experiments.

Mice are timid little creatures. They scurry around their environment, not being still long except to eat, and they prefer darkness. A relatively humane way to subject mice to stress is to confine them in a Lucite tube in a well-lit environment for several hours. If you do this for several days, the mice will exhibit changes in their behavior that resemble depression in humans: they don't eat as much and lose weight. They don't sleep well, and their sexual activity is reduced. They are less active; they spend less time running on the wheels in their cages. (Is this sounding familiar?) Neuroscientists have discovered that when these behavioral changes occur, there are also striking changes in neurons in an area of the brain called the *hippocampus*. We know that this part of the brain is a critical center for emotional regulation in humans. As figure 12.1

shows, when one examines the neurons from the hippocampus of a stressed mouse under the microscope, they look pretty different from the neurons of a non-stressed mouse.

A neuron from a stressed animal (B) looks shrunken and stunted compared to one from a non-stressed animal (A). This same experimental stress causes an increase in stress hormone levels in the bloodstream. It turns out that injecting the mouse equivalent of the human stress hormone cortisol into non-stressed rodents produces precisely the same effect in their brains: shrunken neurons, especially in the hippocampus. Taken together, these findings indicate that chronically elevated levels of stress hormones are responsible for the brain damage that experimental stress causes.

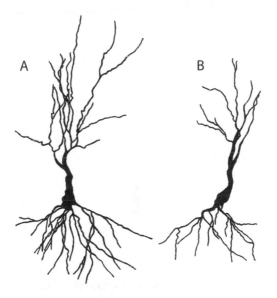

Figure 12.1. The effects of stress on neurons in the hippocampus. A is a representative hippocampal neuron from a control animal, and B is from an animal that was subjected to chronic stress for several hours daily for ten consecutive days. *Source: A. Vyas, R. Mitra, B. S. Shankaranarayana Rao, and S. Chattarji, "Chronic Stress Induces Contrasting Patterns of Dendritic Remodeling in Hippocampal and Amygdaloid Neurons,"* Journal of Neuroscience *22, no. 15 (2002): 6810–18. https://doi.org/10.1523 /JNEUROSCI.22-15-06810.2002. Copyright 2002, Society for Neuroscience.*

But here's the most impressive thing of all: lithium can *prevent* stress-caused damage to brain cells in the mouse's hippocampus. Scientists at Rockefeller University, along with colleagues at other institutions, designed an experiment to investigate whether lithium might protect neurons in the hippocampus from the effects of stress. They took experimental mice and divided them into two groups. For two weeks, they gave lithium to one group but not to the other. Then, they stressed both groups. The picture in figure 12.2 is one of those that's worth a thousand words.

The first cell is from a control animal that was not stressed; it shows a normally developed cell (*A*). Cell *B* is a neuron from a stressed mouse, showing, as expected, a stunted and shrunken cell. *C* is a cell from the hippocampus of a mouse that received lithium for two weeks before and while being subjected to stress.

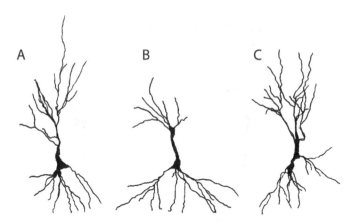

Figure 12.2. Protecting hippocampal neurons from the damaging effects of chronic stress with lithium. *A* is a representative hippocampal neuron from a control animal, *B* is from an animal subjected to twenty-one days of immobilization stress, and *C* is from a stressed animal that had been pretreated with lithium for two weeks before experiencing the stress. *Source: G. Wood, L. Young, L. Reagan, B. Chen, and B. McEwan, "Stress-Induced Structural Remodeling in Hippocampus: Prevention by Lithium Treatment,"* Proceedings of the National Academy of Sciences *101, no. 11 (2004): 3973–78. https://doi.org/10.1073/pnas.0400208101. Copyright 2004, National Academy of Sciences, U.S.A.*

You don't need to be a neuroscientist to see that the cell from the lithium-treated mouse (C) doesn't show the effects of stress. It looks just as healthy as the one from the control animal (A). Lithium has *protected* the brain from the damaging effects of stress.

Results from experiments like these have led to lithium being said to have a *neuroprotective* effect on the brain; it protects the brain from stress-induced damage.

Now, you may be wondering if this means that stress causes bipolar disorder. I can confidently say that the answer to that question is an unequivocal no. We know that stress can be a *trigger* for episodes of illness, especially early in the course of bipolar disorder, but those stressors are acting on vulnerabilities in the brain that appear to be genetic. People who do not have these genetic risks do not develop bipolar symptoms when stressed. It appears that people with bipolar disorder inherit risk genes that make specific brain processes inefficient and subject to breaking down. If you add certain environmental effects—and stress is an important one—on top of these vulnerabilities, the result is a bipolar mood episode.

PICTURING BIPOLAR DISORDER IN THE BRAIN

Brain imaging studies have found that brain areas thought to be important for emotional regulation are smaller in people with bipolar disorder than in people without it. These studies have also demonstrated changes in the activity of and communication between these areas in people with bipolar disorder.

Although we can't see individual brain cells in people with bipolar disorder like we can in experimental animals, we can visualize their brains with MRI (magnetic resonance imaging) and other imaging techniques. These studies have demonstrated what you might expect to see in people if their individual brain cells are damaged and shrunken: several areas of the brain that are important

What about Neuroplasticity?

If you've already been reading other material about mood disorders, you may be wondering why I haven't brought up *neuroplasticity*. Once a concept discussed only among neuroscientists, it now seems to be all the rage. A quick internet search comes up with many websites with recommendations on increasing your neuroplasticity, from "brain exercises" to diets. Let's unpack the word: *neuro-* refers, of course, to the brain and more specifically to neurons; *plasticity* means the ability to be molded and remolded. Neuroplasticity has been defined as the brain's ability to adapt. This adaptation involves rewiring neuronal networks in response to environmental stimuli: neurons make new connections with other neurons and prune old ones. Some links become stronger, others weaker. Areas of the brain constantly rewire themselves to carry out new tasks better and adapt to the continually changing environment. One area of the brain where this process is especially robust is in our friend, the hippocampus.

In this chapter, I've been talking a lot about neurons needing to be "healthy" for the mood control system to work properly, and I've shown you how lithium "protects" neurons. But I could just have easily said that neurons need to have intact neuroplasticity to function normally and that lithium enhances neuroplasticity. An impairment in neuroplasticity appears to be an important aspect of what causes bipolar disorder. Almost all of the treatments for bipolar disorder (and unipolar depression, for that matter) have been shown to enhance neuroplasticity in some way.

in mood control are smaller in people with bipolar disorder than healthy controls. These studies also show that the longer a person has been ill, the more severe this loss of brain tissue becomes. But the good news is that they also show that lithium reverses the process and normalizes the size of these brain areas.

Here is an even more intriguing finding: in a study of healthy young adults who were at high risk for developing bipolar disorder because of a parent with the illness, one of these brain areas was *larger* than average. It's almost as if that area of the brain has bulked up in these at-risk individuals, as if it needed to work overtime to keep them well.

The next questions to ask: What are the neurons in these areas of the brain not doing that they should be doing? Why do these sick cells cause mania and depression?

THE MUSIC OF THE BRAIN

You probably have already learned some things about the brain in science or psychology courses you've taken. You may know that different areas of the brain have different functions. Perhaps you know that there is a language center on the left side of the brain above the ear. There's an area in the back of the brain that processes the information coming from our eyes, and a group of cells deep in the brain that regulates our breathing. There are also areas of the brain that are involved in emotional processing. You've already heard about one, the *hippocampus*. (Like many scientific names for parts of the brain, its name refers to its shape, which early anatomists thought resembled that of a seahorse; *hippocampus* is Greek for "seahorse.") The *amygdala* ("almond") is another, and there are many more.

What you may not have learned about is how different brain areas are connected and work together in complex networks to carry out more complicated tasks like reacting to uncertain situations, learning and remembering, and, yes, emotional processing. The members of these networks are in constant communication with each other, sharing information, giving feedback based on stored memories, sending data back for reprocessing, and so forth.

With MRI it is now possible to measure the activity of brain areas in the networks important for mood regulation. We can now compare their activity levels in people with bipolar disorder to those seen in healthy controls. These studies have demonstrated that certain brain areas are underactive in people with bipolar disorder, while others are on overdrive. The result is that brain networks get out of balance. If you think of normal mood as beautiful music played by an accomplished orchestra, abnormal mood is like a group of musicians who aren't listening to each other, the brass drowning out the violins and the flutes and piccolos coming in too soon. These areas with abnormal activity levels are by and large the same ones that are different in people with bipolar disorder.

These imaging studies have given rise to the idea of *altered connectivity* in specific brain networks as an important cause of mood disorders. The idea is that some brain areas involved in mood regulation are paying too much attention to areas that are the source of strong emotions (the amygdala is one) and not paying enough attention to areas that should regulate their activity.

PUTTING IT ALL TOGETHER

So what causes bipolar disorder? Let's connect the dots: some people inherit abnormal genes or risk genes that endow them with inefficiencies and vulnerabilities in brain systems that regulate mood. Environmental factors, especially stress and the hormonal changes it brings about, act on these vulnerabilities. The result is damaged neurons in brain areas important for mood regulation. This damage disrupts brain networks involved in mood regulation, and the result is a bipolar mood episode.

GENETIC FACTORS

Bipolar disorder is a highly genetic illness, and there appear to be many genes that confer the risk of developing it.

Genetics is the science of heredity, the field that studies the mechanisms by which traits pass from parents to offspring. These include physical traits, like eye color and left-handedness, and also many diseases. It has long been recognized that bipolar disorder exists in clusters within families. In *Manic-Depressive Insanity*, Emil Kraepelin wrote of one family in which "of the ten children of the same parents who were both probably manic-depressive by predisposition, no fewer than seven fell ill the same way." He also noted that "Of the five descendants of the [next] generation, four have already fallen ill."

Genetic Diseases

For some disorders, the links from a specific gene to a particular protein to a trait or disease are easy to follow. Sickle cell anemia is one such disease. People with this disease have an abnormality in the oxygen-carrying molecule in red blood cells, *hemoglobin*. Sickle cell hemoglobin (now called hemoglobin S) differs from normal hemoglobin because of a single misprint in the gene that codes for hemoglobin in people with the disease. Because of this fact, sickle cell anemia is called a *single-gene disease.* We know that several other illnesses are single-gene diseases. These include cystic fibrosis, many forms of hemophilia, and Duchenne muscular dystrophy.

However, bipolar disorder is not one of these single-gene diseases. Like many other common illnesses, such as type 2 diabetes and high blood pressure, bipolar disorder has *complex genetics*. This means that *many* different genes are involved in causing the illness. Geneticists have discovered that many, perhaps dozens, of gene mutations are likely to be involved in determining who develops the illness. Also, each of these mutations may increase the risk of

DNA: The Most Famous Molecule on the Planet

You may have heard the name Gregor Mendel in a high school science class. If so, you know that in experiments with garden pea plants, Mendel discovered the units of inheritance that we now call *genes*. Mendel, and many scientists after him, worked out the rules of inheritance by crossbreeding plants and animals and by observing how human parents transmitted traits to their children. But for a very long time, they were in the dark about how this process worked at the molecular level. Put another way, they didn't know what genes were made of.

It wasn't until the mid-1940s that experiments with bacteria showed that a family of biochemical compounds found in cells, called *nucleic acids*, contained genetic information. In 1953 James Watson, Francis Crick, and Rosalind Franklin published a series of papers in the British scientific journal *Nature* describing the structure of the most important of these compounds: deoxyribonucleic acid (DNA). The modern age of genetics had begun.

DNA molecules are long spiral chains whose links consist of four simpler compounds called *nucleotides*. The four DNA nucleotides—adenine, cytosine, guanine, and thymine (usually abbreviated as A, C, G, and T)—are the elements of an elegantly simple code. Just as you can write out a Morse code version of *Hamlet* using only dots and dashes, you can write out instructions for building hemoglobin, myosin, collagen, or any other protein using As, Cs, Gs, and Ts. That's what DNA does. You can think of the physical structure of a single gene as the section on the DNA molecule that contains the code for one protein.

When the DNA molecule is doing its work in the cell, it is unraveled and stretched out, surrounded by a whole retinue of ultramicroscopic attendants busily reading the coded instructions and making proteins. When it's time for the cell to divide, another set of attendants carefully coil the DNA molecule into a compact cylinder and surround it with protective proteins to form the threadlike structures you may have looked at under the microscope in high school biology: the chromosomes.

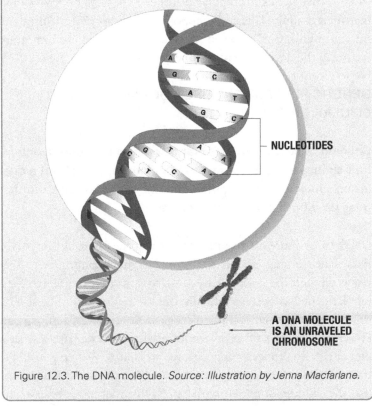

NUCLEOTIDES

A DNA MOLECULE IS AN UNRAVELED CHROMOSOME

Figure 12.3. The DNA molecule. *Source: Illustration by Jenna Macfarlane.*

developing bipolar disorder by just a few percentage points. Only when a "critical mass" or a particular combination of risk genes are present does an individual become ill. Thus, different people with bipolar disorder may have different combinations of risk genes, even though their symptoms are similar. This may explain why individuals vary so widely in their symptoms and their treatment requirements. As you've already read, lithium works quite well for some people but not others. Some people with bipolar disorder can safely take antidepressants, and others cannot. Bipolar disorder's complex genetics are probably a big reason for this. All this complexity also means that there is as yet no reliable genetic test for bipolar disorder.

As you might expect, many of the genes that have been implicated as risk genes for bipolar disorder appear to be involved in neuron signaling. This adds support to the idea that misfires and miscommunication between specific brain centers are important factors in the development of bipolar disorder.

GENETIC RISK FOR CHILDREN OF PARENTS WITH BIPOLAR DISORDER

Children of people with bipolar disorder have about a one-in-four chance of developing a mood disorder and about a one-in-ten chance of developing bipolar disorder. The number goes up if both parents are affected.

Children of individuals with bipolar disorder have an increased risk of developing bipolar disorder. Assigning a number to that risk is difficult for some of the same reasons that the search for a bipolar gene has been so difficult. But the risk seems to be several times that of the general population, in the order of ten percent. However, children of people with bipolar disorder are also at a higher risk for unipolar (depression-only) illness. When you add in this risk, the percentages go up into the high twenties. This means that the children of people with bipolar disorder have about a one-in-four chance of developing some kind of mood disorder and about a one-in-ten chance of developing bipolar disorder.

Individuals with bipolar disorder need to be alert to signs and symptoms of mood disorders in their children and to get them into treatment if such symptoms occur. Although we may be uncertain about the details of the inheritance of bipolar disorder, we are not at all unsure about the importance of early diagnosis and treatment.

Key Takeaways

❖ *By investigating the effects of lithium on the brain, neuroscientists are finding that lithium has a neuroprotective effect that may underlie its efficacy, as well as that of other medications for bipolar disorder.*

❖ *Brain imaging studies have found that brain areas important for emotional regulation are differently sized in people with bipolar disorder compared to healthy controls. These studies have also demonstrated altered connectivity between these areas in people with bipolar disorder.*

❖ *Bipolar disorder runs in families, and children of people with bipolar disorder have about a one-in-four chance of developing a mood disorder and about a one-in-ten chance of developing bipolar disorder. The number goes up if both parents are affected.*

❖ *The genetics of bipolar disorder are complex; dozens of probable risk genes have been identified, but which are most important, what combination is necessary, and how they all interact are all still unknown.*

❖ *There is no reliable genetic test for bipolar disorder.*

CHAPTER 13

How Treatments Work

MEDICATIONS

Medications for bipolar disorder appear to work by enhancing the functioning of neurons in brain circuits involved with mood control. They do this mainly in two ways:

- **By *neuroprotective* mechanisms, best demonstrated in the case of lithium**

- **By triggering new neurons to develop from stem cells in the brain, best seen in antidepressant medications, a process called *neurogenesis***

Some medications appear to work through both of these mechanisms.

As you read in the last chapter, the symptoms of bipolar disorder appear to be caused by problems in the brain networks that control emotional processing and emotional regulation. Those problems, in turn, seem to be caused by injury to neurons in the brain areas that make up these networks. Much of this injury appears to be related to elevated stress hormones such as cortisol. Still, other factors have been implicated as well. Underlying both of these are genetic factors that appear to cause neurons to be susceptible to these damaging effects and subject to breakdown.

What about Serotonin?

Perhaps conspicuous by its absence in this section so far is any discussion of *serotonin*. If you've done other reading about mood disorders, you've almost certainly come across it before. Serotonin is a *neurotransmitter*, one of the brain chemicals neurons use to talk to one another. The electrical impulse that travels through a neuron causes the release of these molecules at the junction between it and neighboring neurons, called a *synapse* (figure 13.1 *inset*). In this book, you've already heard about how various medications change the amount of serotonin and other neurotransmitters in the brain. This effect was discovered relatively early on in research on the effects of antidepressants. For a time, it was believed that abnormal levels of neurotransmitters caused mood disorders, leading to the now old-fashioned term "chemical imbalance" to describe these illnesses. However, it was soon discovered that when experimental animals are given these medications in the lab, neurotransmitter levels go up in their brains within *hours*. It was well known, however, that these medications take *weeks* to work on depression. Hence, the "chemical imbalance" theory started to fall apart almost as soon as it appeared.

We now know that the increase in neurotransmitter levels these medications bring about is just the first step in a cascading series of biochemical effects that eventually results in more profound changes in the brain: the neuro-protective effects and development of new neurons (neurogenesis) that appear to bring about recovery from mood symptoms.

You've already heard about the neuroprotective effects of lithium on cells in the brain areas that are responsible for mood regulation. Other mood stabilizers, such as lamotrigine and valproate, are also thought to have neuroprotective effects.

Antidepressant medications mainly bring about their benefits by triggering new neurons to develop, a process called *neurogenesis*.

For many years, scientists thought that, by the time we are about eighteen months old, our brain has all the neurons we will ever have and that no new neurons will ever develop. That idea has now been thoroughly discredited. We now know that antidepressant medications cause new neurons to develop in—you guessed it—the hippocampus and possibly in other brain areas as well. Animal studies have shown that exposure to several weeks of antidepressant medication is required for this to occur. Feeding Prozac to lab rats for only a few days doesn't bring about the same effect.

These findings about how antidepressant medications work (their mechanism of action) don't explain why these drugs destabilize so many people with bipolar disorder. The fact that they have such a different mechanism of action from lithium may explain why they have such a different and dramatic effect on some individuals.

The atypical antipsychotics appear to operate through both of these mechanisms. They have neuroprotective effects and also trigger hippocampal neurogenesis.

Now that you better understand what medications are doing, several things that you already know about medications will begin to make more sense. First of all, it becomes clear why most medications take weeks or even months to become maximally effective. Getting better from a severe mood episode is not unlike recovering from a broken bone. Cells must heal and regrow, a process that takes time. The chemical signals from medication turn on genes and it takes time for neurons to carry out these genetic orders. The neurons' communicating fibers (called dendrites and

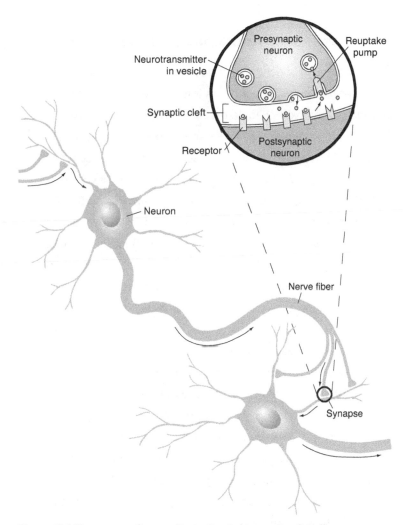

Figure 13.1. The neuron. *Source: Illustration by Jacqueline Schaffer.*

axons) must lengthen, and stem cells must develop into mature neurons and into the support cells for neurons (glial cells). This all takes time. Just as healing from a bone fracture can't be hurried, neither can the healing processes that medications for bipolar disorder bring about.

Fast-Acting Antidepressant Treatments

You may be wondering how treatment with ketamine and esketamine (Spravato) fits into this section on how medications work. People receiving these medications often report that they feel better within *hours* of receiving them. This appears to be because these drugs cause a rapid change in one of the primary neurotransmitters involved in the mood regulation network, *glutamate*. This surge in glutamate seems to quickly restore the normal level of communication in the mood regulation network. Then, there is a second growth phase during which other mechanisms kick in to keep the network working normally. By quickly correcting the altered functional connectivity in the network, the glutamate surge quickly relieves depression symptoms. The second phase keeps it that way.

A new group of medications called *neurosteroids* also have been found to improve mood rapidly. The first of these, brexanolone (Zulresso), was approved to treat postpartum depression in 2019, and others are in development. Like ketamine, these drugs appear to rapidly change the balance of a critical neurotransmitter, *gamma-aminobutyric acid* (GABA), and people notice an improvement in mood within hours rather than weeks.

The older antidepressants eventually bring about similar changes, but because they work through more indirect mechanisms, their benefit takes much longer to become apparent.

B. Luscher, M. Feng, and S. J. Jefferson, "Antidepressant Mechanisms of Ketamine: Focus on GABAergic Inhibition," *Advances in Pharmacology* 89 (2020): 43–78. https://doi.org/10.1016/bs.apha.2020.03.002.

BRAIN STIMULATION TREATMENTS

Brain stimulation treatments directly target areas of the brain that are under- or overactive in mood disorders and use electrical impulses to *upregulate* or *downregulate* neuronal activity in those areas.

In the last chapter, you read about *altered connectivity* in the brain networks involved in mood regulation. Brain stimulation treatments appear to work through similar mechanisms as medications, stimulating biochemical processes that result in neurons becoming more active.

Transcranial magnetic stimulation (TMS) has the advantage of targeting an area on the surface of the brain that neuroimaging research has shown to be underactive in people with depression. TMS devices deliver magnetic impulses directly to this area, called the left *dorsolateral prefrontal cortex*. The activity in this area of the brain is *upregulated*—that is, triggered to be more active—and the normal activity level is restored.

The mechanism of action of *electroconvulsive therapy* (ECT) is less well understood. It has been shown that a seizure raises the levels of many brain chemicals, but other bodily systems, including that system involved in the release of cortisol by the adrenal glands, are affected as well. It's been suggested that ECT works *both* by stimulating growth in neurons (as medications do) *and* by upregulating activity in important brain centers. This dual-action mechanism may explain ECT's high degree of effectiveness compared to most other treatments.

COUNSELING AND PSYCHOTHERAPY

People with bipolar disorder report that therapy helps them understand themselves and their illness better and allows them to take charge of their recovery and take better care of themselves.

So far, this section on how treatments work has focused entirely on medical interventions and the changes they bring about in brain functioning. So how can simply *talking* make things better? How this happens on the cellular level is more mysterious, but some of the same forces appear to be at work.

But explaining how psychotherapy is helpful in terms of biology misses an important point—the human element (table 13.1).

A study from 2018 interviewed thirty young adults with bipolar disorder who had been in a psychotherapy research project. Interviewers asked them to describe *how* psychotherapy had been helpful for them. Three main themes emerged:

• Psychotherapy helped these young people understand themselves better. They were more able to understand and accept their strengths and weaknesses, personal preferences, and personality traits. Also, they learned how these factors impacted their relationships. Crucially, therapy helped them to separate who they are when they are healthy from who they were when they were ill. That is, they were better able to appreciate what were normal feelings and what were symptoms of illness.

• Therapy helped them to understand how having bipolar disorder changed their self-image in ways they hadn't realized. Importantly, they came to see themselves as a person with an illness but not *defined* by their illness.

• Therapy helped them learn about their own unique experience of the illness, their triggers, early signs of mood instability, and what to do about them. They learned how to take better care of themselves.

In Their Own Words:
How Psychotherapy Helps

■ "I think the thing I took away from the therapy was an understanding of how things really affect me—the illness is as individual as the person. [It] made me aware of weak points and [know to] work around these."

■ "I learned how to live with BD and that I could overcome it . . . It didn't have to be a disability . . . at first it was a disability, but it was part of me and I needed to learn how to live with it."

■ "When I first came here, I was taking lots of drugs and drinking lots and had no idea how to deal with my feelings. But now I know."

■ "I realized the problem's not me—it's not my fault but it's because of something that I have. But I learned that it is something that can be managed. Otherwise I would blame everything on myself—I know now there are things I can do to manage it."

■ "[Therapy] was helpful because I got to understand bipolar disorder. Because before I didn't really understand it and what it meant for me . . . the things that helped most were the strategies—routines, turning TV off in the bedroom, recognizing things before they get too bad."

M. Crowe and M. Inder, "Staying Well with Bipolar Disorder: A Qualitative Analysis of Five-Year Follow-Up Interviews with Young People," *Journal of Psychiatric and Mental Health Nursing* 25, no. 4 (2018): 236–44. https://doi.org/10.1111/jpm.12455.

Table 13.1. Benefits of psychotherapy for bipolar disorder

Studies have shown that it results in . . .

Fewer relapses
Increased mood stability
Reduced anxiety
Reduced hopelessness
Improved medication adherence
Improved social functioning and employment

Source: Steven Jones, "Psychotherapy of Bipolar Disorder: A Review," *Journal of Affective Disorders* 80, nos. 2–3 (2004): 101–14. https://doi.org/10.1016/S0165 -0327(03)00111-3.

MOOD HYGIENE

Good mood hygiene diminishes the harmful effects of factors that increase mood instability:

- **Healthy sleep habits help maintain the normal functioning of brain networks that are disrupted by sleep deprivation.**

- **Stress management techniques reduce the level of cortisol and other stress hormones in the body, as well as the effects of inflammation on neurons.**

Avoiding Sleep Deprivation

As you learned in chapter 9, an essential element of mood hygiene is avoiding sleep deprivation. You may remember the study in which healthy volunteers entered an artificial environment that disrupted their sleep-wake cycle: the more out of sync their cycle became, the worse their mood became. More recently, imaging studies have made it possible to see what's happening in the brain when people are deprived of sleep. These studies show that sleep deprivation causes disrupted communication within the mood control network of the brain in healthy individuals in a strikingly similar pattern to that seen in people with bipolar disorder. Some of the same brain areas that are under- or over-active in people with bipolar symptoms become under- or over-active when healthy subjects are deprived of sleep. What's more, the emotional changes that these healthy volunteers experience include irritability, emotional volatility, and an increase in emotional reactivity—symptoms that are not so different from those of mania.

Sleep deprivation also triggers the release of stress hormones like cortisol, which you've already learned is bad for neurons—especially neurons in that important mood control center, the hippocampus. Another negative influence on brain functioning that I've not discussed so far is inflammation. If you've ever suffered a broken bone, you know that the area around the break becomes swollen and often gets hot and red. An infected cut is swollen and red and may leak pus. These changes are the result of inflammation. Inflammation is the result of an activated immune system, usually triggered by an injury or infection. The inflammatory response includes the activation of white blood cells, which produce an array of substances called inflammatory proteins. These proteins usually are involved in marking bacterial invaders for destruction by the immune system and removing dead cells. However, a number of things can cause high levels of these proteins in the absence of infection. These include obesity, poor diet, and, yes, sleep deprivation. Just as chronically elevated stress hormones are harmful to neurons, chronically elevated inflammatory proteins have similar effects.

Sleep deprivation, then, causes mood instability in all kinds of ways: directly impacting signaling and connectivity in the mood control network and increasing the levels of stress hormones and inflammatory proteins in the bloodstream—bad news all around.

What can you do about all this? *Maintain good sleep hygiene!*

Managing Stress

If you've read the last chapter carefully enough, you can probably skip this section—or maybe even write it yourself. You now know that both physical and emotional stresses that persist for too long cause elevated stress hormones like cortisol, which are directly damaging to important neurons involved in maintaining normal signaling and connectivity in the brain's mood control network, to be released.

What can you do about this? Put into action all those healthy practices that your mother and high school health teacher tried to instill in you: a healthy diet, regular exercise, cutting down or cutting out alcohol and nicotine, and the rest of those health-promoting habits that I listed in chapter 9. You might want to reread that chapter right now—not only will it make more sense the second time around, but the importance of mood hygiene will be so much more apparent now that you know something about the causes of bipolar disorder.

Why Zebras Don't Get Ulcers

Neuroscientist Robert Sapolsky highlighted the difference between the stress response in humans and other animals in a book about the role of stress in health and disease called *Why Zebras Don't Get Ulcers*. The book title refers to the fact that when a grazing zebra spots a lion on the edge of the jungle, its stress response kicks in at full force and the animal bounds off at breakneck speed. If the zebra is fast enough and lucky enough, it escapes the hungry lion. It then simply resumes eating, as calm and tranquil as if nothing had happened, with bodily functions quickly returning to baseline. Other than the sight of a lion, there isn't much that brings on the stress response in zebras, because zebras don't have the cognitive capacity to worry.

In the book, Sapolsky illustrates how different humans' stress response is from that of animals like the zebra. In animals, the stress response is either active or inactive; the system is either "on" or "off." But in humans (and the animals most closely related to them), elements of the stress response can be active for much more extended periods. Humans have the capacity to worry about things. "We humans can be stressed by things that simply make no sense to zebras . . . It is not a general mammalian trait to become anxious about mortgages or the Internal Revenue Service, about public speaking or fears of what you say in a job interview, about the inevitability of death." Nevertheless, these very un-zebralike sources of stress activate many of the same physiological responses in the human body as a zebra's sighting of a lion or a hiker's encounter with a bear. This activation results in increases in the stress hormone cortisol that can last for weeks or months at a time.

Robert Sapolsky, *Why Zebras Don't Get Ulcers*, 3rd ed. (New York: Holt Paperbacks, 2004), 7.

Key Takeaways

❖ *Medications help people with bipolar disorder because of their neuroprotective effects on neurons or by triggering new neurons to develop in mood centers of the brain. Both of these mechanisms can be said to increase neuroplasticity.*

❖ *Brain stimulation treatments help by directly stimulating under- or overactive brain areas to restore the normal balance of activity in the mood regulation network of the brain.*

❖ *Psychotherapy helps people with bipolar disorder to better understand themselves and their illness.*

❖ *Mood hygiene addresses environmental factors that can trigger mood episodes and mitigates their destabilizing effects.*

PART V

Putting It All Together

❖Much progress has been made in understanding the causes of bipolar disorder, and the progress is continuing at a dizzying pace.

A short final chapter looks into the future and describes some of the exciting possibilities that researchers hope will help us better understand, diagnose, and treat bipolar disorder, perhaps prevent it from developing, and, yes, maybe even one day cure this illness.

CHAPTER 14

Summing Up and Looking Ahead

We are making enormous progress in the field of psychiatry. The diagnosis of bipolar disorder and other psychiatric illnesses is becoming more accurate all the time. The available treatments for these illnesses are more effective, and there are more of them than ever before. In the past, treatment advances came about mostly by accident and through trial and error, not because of a scientific understanding of the causes of this illness. This is no longer the case.

The most dramatic developments have come from the field of *neuroscience*, the study of the biology and chemistry of the brain and nervous system. At the beginning of the twentieth century, the physical and psychiatric examination of people with brain disorders and the microscopic study of brain tissue obtained from them after death were the only available methods to investigate the diseases of the brain. Animal experiments complemented these studies, but this work resulted in only the vaguest outline of the organization of brain function. The location of brain areas important for speech, movement, vision, and so forth were discovered. Still, psychiatric illnesses remained so mysterious that theories having nothing to do with biology—theories such as psychoanalysis—were the only ones that seemed to offer any hope of understanding these problems.

By the beginning of the twenty-first century, however, one breakthrough after another came about. More powerful electron microscopes allowed the visualization of synapses and other cellular structures, and sophisticated chemical probes allowed scientists to work out the mechanisms by which neurons develop and communicate with each other. Understanding continues to accumulate concerning the fine details of how neurons link to and communicate with each other and how these processes can go awry.

New technologies for brain imaging have allowed scientists to see the brain at work in living people for the first time. We now have imaging techniques that can trace changes in blood flow within the brain, locate areas that are over- or underactive, and detect abnormally high or low levels of brain chemicals. This information reveals how the interplay of activity between different brain areas is essential in regulating mood. With these new techniques, we can see how these networks operate differently in a person with a mood disorder compared to a person who does not have the condition. Perhaps an even more significant benefit will result because we can now observe the changes in the brain when a person receives treatment and is beginning to feel well again.

Another of the innovative scientific disciplines advancing the search for causes and better treatments is the field of *genetics*. Here again, it is the development of new biochemical methods and molecular probes that have made this new research possible. With the announcement that the Human Genome Project had mapped all of the genetic material in the human chromosomes, a new era in the understanding of genetics began. The discovery of new genes is announced every day, and it is only a matter of time before geneticists unravel the genetic mechanisms of mood disorders.

The first genetic approach to pay off in changing treatment is likely to be *pharmacogenomics*, the field within genetics that investigates genetic factors associated with responses to particular pharmaceuticals rather than disease risk. Pharmacogenomics promises that therapeutic agents can be rationally selected based on a person's genetic profile rather than the trial-and-error process people must now endure. In the not-too-distant future, a blood test will show whether lithium or valproate or lamotrigine or some as yet undiscovered drug will be the best treatment for a particular individual with bipolar disorder. A blood test may be able to identify people with bipolar disorder who can safely take an antidepressant.

As the genetic basis of mood disorders is discovered, it may turn out that our classification system for them is all wrong. We may need a whole new diagnostic approach for psychiatric illnesses, perhaps one based on the genes involved in individual people. Instead of "bipolar disorder II," we may be diagnosing people with something like "DISC I disorder," a diagnostic label derived from the name of a gene.

These different fields are closing in on the causes and mechanisms of mood disorders from different directions. As these enterprises advance, they will begin to inform each other—advances in one field will lead to advances in the other. The discovery that a gene for a particular protein is linked to a mood disorder will tell neuroscientists that that protein is important in mood regulation. The discovery of an enzyme in the brain that is important for neurogenesis will tell geneticists to focus on the gene for that enzyme in their studies. Little by little, the whole picture will become increasingly clear.

Skin cells from a simple biopsy can now be transformed into stem cells or even neurons in the laboratory and tested for responses to particular drugs. It will be a while yet before this technique is widely available for individual people. Still, when it is, it will represent the apex of personalized medicine and take much of the guesswork out of treatment.

As our understanding of the biology of mood disorders improves, we get closer to better diagnostic methods and safer and more effective treatments. The number of new medications continues to grow and many more new pharmaceuticals are "in the pipeline," some of them based on clues about the biological causes of these illnesses. The era of finding new medications essentially by accident is coming to a close; researchers are already designing treatments more effectively and rationally. More sophisticated use of nonpharmaceutical therapies such as transcranial magnetic stimulation may make it possible to use lower doses of medications or help medications work more quickly.

As we take the step from isolating genes to determining the function of those genes, gene therapy is possible: repairing the code in the DNA that causes mood disorders. The obstacles to be overcome before we can look for this type of cure are still daunting. Stem-cell infusions are being used to treat a variety of neurological illnesses. As scientists are learning more and more about the neurological basis of bipolar disorder, a cure might be possible.

As we identify the mechanisms by which illness develops and the genetic vulnerabilities that put individuals at risk, another exciting possibility emerges: *prevention*. Genetic data and a better understanding of what triggers the condition may allow the development of programs to prevent the illness from developing in individuals at higher risk for a particular disorder.

So there is a good reason to expect great strides in our ability to diagnose and effectively treat bipolar disorder. But we have *already* made great strides—individuals with bipolar disorder must not let denial or fear stand in the way of taking advantage of the excellent treatments that are now available. Ignorance is no excuse, either. Support organizations provide up-to-date information about bipolar disorder through newsletters, brochures, websites, and, most importantly, the support groups they sponsor (see the list of resources that follows this chapter). With the ever-growing number of online resources now available, anyone with access to a computer can get the latest information on new pharmaceuticals and other treatments with the click of a mouse.

People with bipolar disorder frequently ask me, "Will I have to take medication for the rest of my life?" I always tell them that no one knows the answer to that question because no one knows what the treatment of mood disorders might be like in the future. Pediatricians practicing in the 1930s probably could not have imagined that vaccines would one day practically eliminate diphtheria, polio, measles, and other childhood diseases—the common, frequently crippling, and sometimes fatal illnesses they diagnosed so often in their patients but were so helpless to treat. The astonishing developments in neuroscience, brain imaging, and genetics hold just as much promise for people afflicted with mood disorders. There is every reason to expect that the time is not too far off when treatments for bipolar disorder will be more effective than we can now imagine.

Suggested Reading

Jahren, Hope. *Lab Girl.* New York: Alfred A. Knopf, 2016.
Who knew trees were so amazing? Written by a brilliant, award-winning scientist who happens to suffer from bipolar disorder. Not your typical bipolar memoir, this book centers more on the struggles of being a woman in science and the author's deep knowledge of the lives of trees, which she relates with infectious enthusiasm. Professor Jahren's brief discussions of her very severe bouts of illness are little more than side notes—as they should be.

Jamison, Kay Redfield. *An Unquiet Mind: A Memoir of Moods and Madness.* New York: Vintage Books, 1996.
A powerful and moving narrative written with grace and wit by an international expert on the illness who suffers from it herself. This treasure of a book contains some of the most engrossing and vivid descriptions of the experience of bipolar disorder ever written. A must-read for anyone touched by bipolar disorder.

Kraepelin, Emil. *Manic-Depressive Insanity and Paranoia.* Translated by R. M. Barclay. Edited by G. M. Robertson. 1921; reprint, New York: Arno Press, 1976.
Many college and university libraries have a copy of this book, and digital versions are readily available online. Arguably the very first textbook on the illness ever written, it is definitely worth reading.

Mondimore, Francis Mark. *Bipolar Disorder: A Guide for You and Your Family.* 4th ed. Baltimore: Johns Hopkins University Press, 2020.

OK, I'm biased in favor of this one. But if reading this book has left you wanting more information, pick up its big brother, which is more detailed and comprehensive.

"An essential guide for patients and their loved ones navigating the challenges of a bipolar illness. Full of helpful examples and straightforward explanations, the book is an easy and necessary read. I highly recommend it." —Patricia Dill Rinvelt, executive director, National Network of Depression Centers.

Noonan, Susan J. *Take Control of Your Depression: Strategies to Help You Feel Better Now.* Baltimore: Johns Hopkins University Press, 2018.

This slim volume is packed with truly helpful advice about managing the symptoms of depression, informed by the author's own struggle with a depressive illness as well as her expertise as a physician and background in public health. Dr. Noonan doesn't just offer suggestions; she also lays out exercises and lifestyle rec-ommendations that are concise and eminently practical. All are presented simply, compassionately, and in small, realistic steps that recognize how difficult it is for a person with depression to get things done.

References

Preface

Dagani, J., G. Signorini, O. Nielssen, M. Bani, A. Pastore, G. de Girolamo, and M. Large. "Meta-analysis of the Interval between the Onset and Management of Bipolar Disorder." *Canadian Journal of Psychiatry / Revue canadienne de psychiatrie* 62, no. 4 (2017): 247–58. https:// doi.org/ 10.1177/ 0706743716656607.

"National Survey of NDMDA Members Finds Long Delay in Diagnosis of Manic-Depressive Illness." In "News and Notes," *Hospital and Community Psychiatry* 44, no. 8 (1993): 800–801.

Chapter 1

Kraepelin, E. *Manic-Depressive Insanity and Paranoia*. Translated by R. M. Barclay. Edited by G. M. Robertson (1921; reprint, New York: Arno Press, 1976), 31. This is a translation of volumes 3 and 4 of the eighth edition (1913) of Kraepelin's textbook (in German) *Psychiatrie*, which originally appeared in 1896.

Chapter 2

Baek, J. H., D. Y. Park, J. Choi, J. S. Kim, J. S. Choi, K. Ha, J. S. Kwon, D. Lee, and K. S. Hong. "Differences between Bipolar I and Bipolar II Disorders in Clinical Features, Comorbidity, and Family History." *Journal of Affective Disorders* 131, nos. 1–3 (2011): 59–67. https:// doi.org/ 10.1016/ j.jad.2010.11.020.

Cochran, A. L., M. G. McInnis, and D. B. Forger. "Data-Driven Classification of Bipolar I Disorder from Longitudinal Course of Mood." *Translational Psychiatry* 6, no. 10 (2016): e912. https:// doi.org/ 10.1038/ tp.2016.166.

Coryell, W., N. C. Andreasen, J. Endicott, and M. Keller. "The Significance of Past Mania or Hypomania in the Course and Outcome of Major Depression." *American Journal of Psychiatry* 144, no. 3 (1987): 309–15. https:// doi.org/10.1176/ajp.144.3.309.

Judd, L. L., H. S. Akiskal, P. J. Schettler, J. Endicott, J. Maser, D. A. Solomon, A. C. Leon, J. A. Rice, and M. B. Keller. "The Long-Term Natural History of the Weekly Symptomatic Status of Bipolar I Disorder." *Archives of General Psychiatry* 59, no. 6 (2002): 530–37. https:// doi.org/10.1001/archpsyc.59.6.530.

Merikangas, K. R., R. Jin, J.-P. He, R. C. Kessler, S. Lee, N. A. Sampson, M. C. Viana, et al. "Prevalence and Correlates of Bipolar Spectrum Disorder in the World Mental Health Survey Initiative." *Archives of General Psychiatry* 68, no. 3 (2011): 241–51. https:// doi.org/10.1001/archgenpsychiatry.2011.12.

Perugi, G., E. Hantouche, G. Vannucchi, and O. Pinto. "Cyclothymia Reloaded: A Reappraisal of the Most Misconceived Affective Disorder." *Journal of Affective Disorders* 183 (2015): 119–33. https:// doi.org/10.1016/j.jad.2015.05.004.

Van Meter, A., E. A. Youngstrom, C. Demeter, and R. L. Findling. "Examining the Validity of Cyclothymic Disorder in a Youth Sample: Replication and Extension." *Journal of Abnormal Child Psychology* 41, no. 3 (2013): 367–78. https:// doi.org/10.1007/s10802-012-9680-1.

Winokur, G., P. J. Clayton, and T. Reich, *Manic-Depressive Illness* (St. Louis: C. V. Mosby, 1969). Quoted in F. K. Goodwin and K. R. Jamison, *Manic-Depressive Illness* (New York: Oxford University Press, 1990), 141.

Chapter 3

Berk, M., D. L. Copolov, O. D., K. Lu, S. Jeavons, I. Schapkaitz, M. Anderson-Hunt, and A. I. Bush. "N-Acetyl Cysteine for Depressive Symptoms in Bipolar Disorder—a Double-Blind Randomized Placebo-Controlled Trial." *Biological Psychiatry* 64, no. 6 (2008): 468–75. https:// doi.org/10.1016/j.biopsych.2008.04.022.

Berk, M., O. Dean, S. M. Cotton, C. S. Gama, F. Kapczinski, B. S. Fernandes, K. Kohlmann, et al. "The Efficacy of N-Acetylcysteine as an Adjunctive Treatment in Bipolar Depression: An Open Label Trial." *Journal of Affective Disorders* 135, nos. 1–3 (2011): 389–94. https:// doi.org/10.1016/j.jad.2011.06.005.

Bowden, C. L., J. R. Calabrese, G. Sachs, L. N. Yatham, S. A. Asghar, M. Hompland, P. Montgomery, N. Earl, T. M. Smoot, and J. DeVeaugh-Geiss (Lamictal 606 Study Group). "A Placebo-Controlled 18-Month Trial of Lamotrigine and Lithium Maintenance Treatment in Recently Manic or Hypomanic Patients with Bipolar I Disorder." *Archives of General Psychiatry* 60, no. 4 (2003): 392–400. https:// doi.org/ 10.1001/ archpsyc.60.4.392.

Calabrese, J. R., C. L. Bowden, G. Sachs, L. N. Yatham, K. Behnke, O. P. Mehtonen, P. Montgomery, et al. "A Placebo-Controlled 18-Month Trial of Lamotrigine and Lithium Maintenance Treatment in Recently Depressed Patients with Bipolar I Disorder." *Journal of Clinical Psychiatry* 64, no. 9 (2003): 1013 24. https:// doi.org/ 10.4088 / jcp.v64n0906.

Calabrese, J. R., J. R. Sullivan, C. L. Bowden, T. Suppes, J. F. Goldberg, G. S. Sachs, M. D. Shelton, F. K. Goodwin, M. A. Frye, and V. Kusumakar. "Rash in Multicenter Trials of Lamotrigine in Mood Disorders: Clinical Relevance and Management." *Journal of Clinical Psychiatry* 63, no. 11 (2002): 1012–19. https:// doi.org/ 10.4088/ jcp .v63n1110.

Centorrino, F., M. J. Albert, J. M. Berry, J. P. Kelleher, V. Fellman, G. Line, A. E. Koukopoulos, J. E. Kidwell, K. V. Fogarty, and R. J. Baldessarini. "Oxcarbazepine: Clinical Experience with Hospitalized Psychiatric Patients." *Bipolar Disorders* 5, no. 5 (2003): 370–74. https:// doi.org/ 10.1034/ j.1399-5618.2003.00047.x.

Goldberg, J. F., K. E. Burdick, and C. J. Endick. "Preliminary Randomized, Double-Blind, Placebo-Controlled Trial of Pramipexole Added to Mood Stabilizers for Treatment-Resistant Bipolar Depression." *American Journal of Psychiatry* 161, no. 3 (2004): 564–66. https:// doi.org/ 10.1176/ appi.ajp.161.3.564.

Lerer, B., N. Moore, E. Meyendorff, S. R. Cho, and S. Gershon. "Carbamazepine versus Lithium in Mania: A Double-Blind Study." *Journal of Clinical Psychiatry* 48, no. 3 (1987): 89–93.

Macritchie, K. A., J. R. Geddes, J. Scott, D. R. Haslam, and G. M. Goodwin. "Valproic Acid, Valproate, and Divalproex in the Maintenance Treatment of Bipolar Disorder." Cochrane Database of Systematic Reviews, no. 3 (2001): art. no. CD003196. https:// doi.org/ 10.1002/ 14651858.CD003196.

Moore, G. J., B. M. Cortese, D. A. Glitz, C. Zajac-Benitez, J. A. Quiroz, T. W. Uhde, W. C. Drevets, and H. K. Manji. "A Longitudinal Study of the Effects of Lithium Treatment on Prefrontal and Subgenual

Prefrontal Gray Matter Volume in Treatment-Responsive Bipolar
Disorder Patients." *Journal of Clinical Psychiatry* 70, no. 5 (2009):
699–705. https://doi.org/10.4088/JCP.07m03745.

Schou, M. "Forty Years of Lithium Treatment." *Archives of General
Psychiatry* 54, no. 1 (1997): 9–13. https://doi.org/10.1001
/archpsyc.1997.01830130013002.

Shorter, Edward. "The History of Lithium Therapy." *Bipolar
Disorders* 11, suppl. 2 (2009): 4–9. https://doi.org/10.1111
/j.1399-5618.2009.00706.x.

Chapter 4

Baptista, T., N. M. Kin, S. Beaulieu, and E. A. de Baptista. "Obesity
and Related Metabolic Abnormalities during Antipsychotic
Drug Administration: Mechanisms, Management, and Research
Perspectives." *Pharmacopsychiatry* 35, no. 6 (2002): 205–19.
https://doi.org/10.1055/s-2002-36391.

Calabrese, J. R., S. E. Kimmel, M. J. Woyshville, D. J. Rapport, C. J.
Faust, P. A. Thompson, and H. Y. Meltzer. "Clozapine for Treatment-
Refractory Mania." *American Journal of Psychiatry* 153, no. 6 (1996):
759–64. https://doi.org/10.1176/ajp.153.6.759.

Hochman, E., A. Krivoy, A. Schaffer, A. Weizman, and A. Valevski.
"Antipsychotic Adjunctive Therapy to Mood Stabilizers and
1-Year Rehospitalization Rates in Bipolar Disorder: A Cohort
Study." *Bipolar Disorders* 18, no. 8 (2016): 684–91. https://doi
.org/10.1111/bdi.12459.

Ray, W. A., C. P. Chung, K. T. Murray, K. Hall, and C. M. Stein.
"Atypical Antipsychotic Drugs and the Risk of Sudden Cardiac
Death." *New England Journal of Medicine* 360, no. 3 (2009): 225–35.
https://doi.org/10.1056/NEJMoa0806994.

Sachs, G. S., A. A. Nierenberg, J. R. Calabrese, L. B. Marangell, S. R.
Wisniewski, L. Gyulai, E. S. Friedman, et al. "Effectiveness of
Adjunctive Antidepressant Treatment for Bipolar Depression." *New
England Journal of Medicine* 356, no. 17 (2007): 1711–22. https://doi
.org/10.1056/NEJMoa064135.

Chapter 5

Bauer, M. S., P. C. Whybrow, and A. Winokur. "Rapid Cycling Bipolar
Affective Disorder I: Association with Grade I Hypothyroidism."

Archives of General Psychiatry 47, no. 5 (1990): 427–32. https://doi.org/10.1001/archpsyc.1990.01810170027005.

Berk, M., O. Dean, S. M. Cotton, C. S. Gama, F. Kapczinski, B. S. Fernandes, K. Kohlmann, et al. "The Efficacy of N-Acetylcysteine as an Adjunctive Treatment in Bipolar Depression: An Open Label Trial." *Journal of Affective Disorders* 135, nos. 1–3 (2011): 389–94. https://doi.org/10.1016/j.jad.2011.06.005.

Cole, D. P., M. E. Thase, A. G. Mallinger, J. C. Soares, J. F. Luther, D. J. Kupfer, and E. Frank. "Slower Treatment Response in Bipolar Depression Predicted by Lower Pretreatment Thyroid Function." *American Journal of Psychiatry* 159, no. 1 (2002): 116–21. https://doi.org/10.1176/appi.ajp.159.1.116.

Dündar, Y., A. Boland, J. Strobl, S. Dodd, A. Haycox, A. Bagust, J. Bogg, R. Dickson, and T. Walley. "Newer Hypnotic Drugs for the Short-Term Management of Insomnia: A Systematic Review and Economic Evaluation." *Health Technology Assessment* 8, no. 24 (2004): iii–x. https://doi.org/10.3310/hta8240.

Keck Jr., P. E., J. R. Strawn, and S. L. McElroy. "Pharmacologic Treatment Considerations in Co-occurring Bipolar and Anxiety Disorders." *Journal of Clinical Psychiatry* 67, suppl. 1 (2006): 8–15.

Sarris, J., D. Mischoulon, and I. Schweitzer. "Omega-3 for Bipolar Disorder: Meta-analyses of Use in Mania and Bipolar Depression." *Journal of Clinical Psychiatry* 73, no. 1 (2012): 81–6. https://doi.org/10.4088/JCP.10r06710.

Shelton, R. C., M. B. Keller, A. Gelenberg, D. L. Dunner, R. Hirschfeld, M. E. Thase, J. Russell, et al. "Effectiveness of St. John's Wort in Major Depression: A Randomized Controlled Trial." *Journal of the American Medical Association* 285, no. 15 (2001): 1978–86. https://doi.org/10.1001/jama.285.15.1978.

Xie, Z., F. Chen, W. A. Li, X. Geng, C. Li, X. Meng, Y. Feng, W. Liu, and F. Yu. "A Review of Sleep Disorders and Melatonin." *Neurological Research* 39, no. 6 (2017): 559–65. https://doi.org/10.1080/01616412.2017.1315864.

Chapter 6

Brus, O., P. Nordanskog, U. Båve, Y. Cao, Å. Hammar, M. Landén, J. Lundberg, and A. Nordenskjöld. "Subjective Memory Immediately Following Electroconvulsive Therapy." *Journal of Electroconvulsive Therapy* 33, no. 2 (2017): 96–103. https://doi.org/10.1097/YCT.0000000000000377.

George, M. S., E. M. Wasserman, T. A. Kimbrell, J. T. Little, W. E. Williams, A. L. Danielson, B. D. Greenberg, M. Hallett, and R. M. Post. "Mood Improvement following Daily Left Prefrontal Repetitive Transcranial Magnetic Stimulation in Patients with Depression: A Placebo-Controlled Crossover Trial." *American Journal of Psychiatry* 154, no. 12 (1997): 1752–56. https://doi.org/10.1176/ajp.154.12.1752.

Vallance, M. "The Experience of Electro-convulsive Therapy by a Practising Psychiatrist." *British Journal of Psychiatry* 111 (1965): 365–67.

Chapter 7

Goldstein, T. R., R. K. Fersch-Podrat, M. Rivera, D. A. Axelson, J. Merranko, H. Yu, D. A. Brent, and B. Birmaher. "Dialectical Behavior Therapy for Adolescents with Bipolar Disorder: Results from a Pilot Randomized Trial." *Journal of Child and Adolescent Psychopharmacology* 25, no. 2 (2015): 140–9. https://doi.org/10.1089/cap.2013.0145.

Ives-Deliperi, V. L., F. Howells, D. J. Stein, E. M. Meintjes, and N. Horn. "The Effects of Mindfulness-Based Cognitive Therapy in Patients with Bipolar Disorder: A Controlled Functional MRI Investigation." *Journal of Affective Disorders* 150, no. 3 (2013): 1152–57. https://doi.org/10.1016/j.jad.2013.05.074.

Kanas, Nick. "Group Psychotherapy with Bipolar Patients: A Review and Synthesis." *International Journal of Group Psychotherapy* 43, no. 3 (1993): 321–33. https://doi.org/10.1080/00207284.1993.11732596.

Pollack, L. E. "Content Analysis of Groups for Inpatients with Bipolar Disorder." *Applied Nursing Research* 6, no. 1 (1993): 19–27. https://doi.org/10.1016/s0897-1897(05)80038-2.

Salcedo, S., A. K. Gold, S. Sheikh, P. H. Marcus, A. A. Nierenberg, T. Deckersbach, and L. G. Sylvia. "Empirically Supported Psychosocial Interventions for Bipolar Disorder: Current State of the Research." *Journal of Affective Disorders* 201 (2016): 203–14. https://doi.org/10.1016/j.jad.2016.05.018.

Scott, Jan. "Psychotherapy for Bipolar Disorder." *British Journal of Psychiatry* 167, no. 5 (1995): 581–88. https://doi.org/10.1192/bjp.167.5.581.

Soo, S. A., Z. W. Zhang, S. J. Khong, J. E. W. Low, V. S. Thambyrajah, S. H. B. T. Alhabsyi, Q. H. Chew, et al. "Randomized Controlled Trials of Psychoeducation Modalities in the Management of Bipolar

Disorder: A Systematic Review." *Journal of Clinical Psychiatry* 79, no. 3 (2018): 17r11750. https://doi.org/10.4088/JCP.17r11750.

Chapter 8

Cakir, S., O. Yazici, and R. M. Post. "Decreased Responsiveness following Lithium Discontinuation in Bipolar Disorder: A Naturalistic Observation Study." *Psychiatry Research* 247, no. 1 (2017): 305–9. https://doi.org/10.1016/j.psychres.2016.11.046.

Hammen, C., and M. Gitlin. "Stress Reactivity in Bipolar Patients and Its Relation to Prior History of Disorder." *American Journal of Psychiatry* 154, no. 6 (1997): 856–57. https://doi.org/10.1176/ajp.154.6.856.

Hunt, G. E., G. S. Malhi, M. Cleary, H. M. X. Lai, and T. Sitharthan. "Prevalence of Comorbid Bipolar and Substance Use Disorders in Clinical Settings, 1990–2015: Systematic review and Meta-analysis." *Journal of Affective Disorders* 206 (2016): 331–49. https://doi.org/10.1016/j.jad.2016.07.011.

Treuer, T., and M. Tohen. "Predicting the Course and Outcome of Bipolar Disorder: A Review." *European Psychiatry* 25, no. 6 (2010): 328–33. https://doi.org/10.1016/j.eurpsy.2009.11.012.

Chapter 9

Boivin, D. B., C. A. Czeisler, D.-J. Dijk, J. F. Duffy, S. Folkard, D. S. Minors, P. Totterdell, and J. M. Waterhouse. "Complex Interaction of the Sleep-Wake Cycle and Circadian Phase Modulates Mood in Healthy Subjects." *Archives of General Psychiatry* 54, no. 2 (1997): 145–52. https://doi.org/10.1001/archpsyc.1997.01830140055010.

Gruber, J., D. J. Miklowitz, A. G. Harvey, E. Frank, D. Kupfer, M. E. Thase, G. S. Sachs, and T. A. Ketter. "Sleep Matters: Sleep Functioning and Course of Illness in Bipolar Disorder." *Journal of Affective Disorders* 134, nos. 1–3 (2011): 416–20. https://doi.org/10.1016/j.jad.2011.05.016.

Prochaska, J. O., and W. F. Velicer. "The Transtheoretical Model of Health Behavior Change." *American Journal of Health Promotion* 12, no. 1 (1997): 38–48. https://doi.org/10.4278/0890-1171-12.1.38.

Rakofsky, J. J., and B. W. Dunlop. "Do Alcohol Use Disorders Destabilize the Course of Bipolar Disorder?" *Journal of Affective Disorders* 145, no. 1 (2013): 1–10. https://doi.org/10.1016/j.jad.2012.06.012.

Chapter 10

Miller, J. N., and D. W. Black. "Bipolar Disorder and Suicide: A Review." *Current Psychiatry Reports* 22, no. 2 (2020): 6. https://doi.org/10.1007/s11920-020-1130-0.

Chapter 12

Crowe, M., and M. Inder. "Staying Well with Bipolar Disorder: A Qualitative Analysis of Five-Year Follow-Up Interviews with Young People." *Journal of Psychiatric and Mental Health Nursing* 25, no. 4 (2018): 236–44. https://doi.org/10.1111/jpm.12455.

Hajek, T., J. Cullis, T. Novak, M. Kopecek, R. Blagdon, L. Propper, P. Stopkova, et al. "Brain Structural Signature of Familial Predisposition for Bipolar Disorder: Replicable Evidence for Involvement of the Right Inferior Frontal Gyrus." *Biological Psychiatry* 73, no. 2 (2013): 144–52. https://doi.org/10.1016/j.biopsych.2012.06.015.

Ikeda, M., T. Saito, K. Kondo, and N. Iwata. "Genome-Wide Association Studies of Bipolar Disorder: A Systematic Review of Recent Findings and Their Clinical Implications." *Psychiatry and Clinical Neurosciences* 72, no. 2 (2018): 52–63. https://doi.org/10.1111/pcn.12611.

Johansson, V., R. Kuja-Halkola, T. D. Cannon, C. M. Hultman, and A. M. Hedman. "A Population-Based Heritability Estimate of Bipolar Disorder—in a Swedish Twin Sample." *Psychiatry Research* 278 (2019), 180–87. https://doi.org/10.1016/j.psychres.2019.06.010.

Phillips, M. L., and H. A. Swartz. "A Critical Appraisal of Neuro-imaging Studies of Bipolar Disorder: Toward a New Conceptualization of Underlying Neural Circuitry and a Road Map for Future Research." *American Journal of Psychiatry* 171, no. 8 (2014): 829–43. https://doi.org/10.1176/appi.ajp.2014.13081008.

Pittenger, C., and R. S. Duman. "Stress, Depression, and Neuro-plasticity: A Convergence of Mechanisms." *Neuropsychopharmacology* 33 (2008): 88–109. https://doi.org/10.1038/sj.npp.1301574.

Chapter 13

Kusumi, I., S. Boku, and Y. Takahashi. "Psychopharmacology of Atypical Antipsychotic Drugs: From the Receptor Binding Profile to Neuroprotection and Neurogenesis." *Psychiatry and Clinical Neurosciences* 69, no. 5 (2015): 243–58. https://doi.org/10.1111/pcn.12242.

Li, M., X. Yao, L. Sun, L. Zhao, W. Xu, H. Zhao, F. Zhao, et al. "Effects of Electroconvulsive Therapy on Depression and Its Potential Mechanism." *Frontiers in Psychology* 11 (2020): 80. https://doi.org/10.3389/fpsyg.2020.00080.

Machado-Vieira, R. "Lithium, Stress, and Resilience in Bipolar Disorder: Deciphering This Key Homeostatic Synaptic Plasticity Regulator." *Journal of Affective Disorders* 233 (2018): 92–9. https://doi.org/10.1016/j.jad.2017.12.026.

Palagini, L., C. H. Bastien, D. Marazziti, J. G. Ellis, and D. Riemann. "The Key Role of Insomnia and Sleep Loss in the Dysregulation of Multiple Systems Involved in Mood Disorders: A Proposed Model." *Journal of Sleep Research* 28, no. 6 (2019): e12841. https://doi.org/10.1111/jsr.12841.

Planchez, B., A. Surget, and C. Belzung. "Adult Hippocampal Neurogenesis and Antidepressants Effects." *Current Opinion in Pharmacology* 50 (2020): 88–95. https://doi.org/10.1016/j.coph.2019.11.009.

Index

HOPKINS PRESS

HEALTH BOOKS

Bipolar Disorder
A Guide for You and Your Loved Ones, *fourth edition*

Francis Mark Mondimore, MD

The vital resource for people with bipolar disorder and their loved ones, completely updated. **$23.95 pb/eb**

Adolescent Depression
A Guide for Parents, *second edition*

Francis Mark Mondimore, MD, and Patrick Kelly, MD

The timely second edition of this bestselling guide will inform and encourage struggling adolescents and their families. **$21.95 pb/eb**

Helping Others with Depression
Words to Say, Things to Do

Susan J. Noonan, MD, MPH

A comprehensive guide to how family members and friends can help someone who has depression. **$19.95 pb/eb**

Take Control of Your Depression
Strategies to Help You Feel Better Now

Susan J. Noonan, MD, MPH

foreword by Jerrold F. Rosenbaum, MD, and Timothy J. Petersen, PhD

Practical, day-to-day ways to manage your depression. **$19.95 pb/eb**

Reconnecting after Isolation
Coping with Anxiety, Depression, Grief, PTSD, and More

Susan J. Noonan, MD, MPH

How to keep calm, carry on, and reconnect during times of social isolation and emotional crisis. **$19.99 pb/eb**

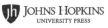 JOHNS HOPKINS UNIVERSITY PRESS

 press.jhu.edu

For more Johns Hopkins Health Books visit **press.jhu.edu**